A STITCH
OF TIME

THE YEAR A BRAIN INJURY CHANGED

MY LANGUAGE AND LIFE

LAUREN MARKS

SIMON & SCHUSTER

NEW YORK LONDON TORONTO SYDNEY NEW DELHI

Simon & Schuster
1230 Avenue of the Americas
New York, NY 10020

First Simon & Schuster hardcover edition May 2017

SIMON & SCHUSTER and colophon are registered
trademarks of Simon & Schuster, Inc.

For information about special discounts for bulk purchases,
please contact Simon & Schuster Special Sales
at 1-866-506-1949 or business@simonandschuster.com.

The Simon & Schuster Speakers Bureau can bring authors to your live event.
For more information or to book an event contact the
Simon & Schuster Speakers Bureau at 1-866-248-3049
or visit our website at www.simonspeakers.com.

Interior design by Ruth Lee-Mui

Manufactured in the United States of America

1   3   5   7   9   10   8   6   4   2

Library of Congress Cataloging-in-Publication Data is available.

ISBN 978-1-4516-9751-3
ISBN 978-1-4516-9761-2 (ebook)

To the fixers and the menders.

To the family who are also my friends.

And to the friends who are also my family.

AUTHOR'S NOTE

On Aphasia and the Unknown Unknowns

Izena duen guztia omen da
(That which has a name exists)
BASQUE PROVERB

Aphasia is something you never see coming. You are born, and as you grow and develop, you acquire words and language skills that partially make you the person you are. But maybe one day, in the span of a single second, you lose it all. The world of words—from poems to prayers, from stories to songs—can suddenly be rendered strange. Though one out of every 250 people is affected by aphasia, the term is not widely known among the general public. I personally knew very little about this condition until I was twenty-seven years old, when an aneurysm ruptured in my brain.

Aphasia can be brought on by all sorts of things, from bike accidents to gunshot wounds, but the most common cause is a stroke. This was how this disorder made its unanticipated entrance into my own life. I suffered a hemorrhagic stroke, a flood in the brain. The path of its damage left its traces in my cells and tissues, which dramatically affected my abilities to speak, read, and write.

Language is wrapped up with our current and remembered sense of identity. We assign certain words to an experience, and some of them become part of our telling and retelling of the event—the script of our lives. But what happens when someone can't access the most intimate and natural parts of their language anymore? When a linguistic template is taken away, the balance of these interactions is bound to change in unexpected ways. Banter between lovers fails to ignite. Inside jokes among friends are observed purely from the outside. The way family members interest, persuade, and comfort one another can all shift. We use words to describe ourselves to others, but also to describe ourselves to ourselves. This makes language and memory often inextricably intertwined.

When writing about a neurological injury, one faces the most basic challenges of memory itself. In *The Seven Sins of Memory*, author Daniel Schacter warns that: "*Past* events are filtered by *current* knowledge," and "people seem almost driven to reconstruct the past to fit what they know in the present." Memory is a constant act of creation. As our versions of ourselves change, our memories change as well, unconsciously adjusting their dimensions to our newest understanding of the world. It is hindsight that provides the illusion of unity in our lives, and hindsight is capable of the most astonishing cognitive trick we possess: transforming the impossible into the inevitable.

Your brain is the organ of perception, so when your brain is damaged, there is a chance that your perceptions are damaged too. After my aneurysm ruptured, I lost the ability to use words effectively, though I wasn't fully aware of that fact at the time. As strange as it may sound, I could understand the spoken language around me, but I often couldn't hear how much my own speech was affected. And it wasn't only my external language. My inner voice was almost mute, too, which meant I couldn't always ask myself questions or sort through my own thoughts. I am aware that this peculiar type of dissonance bleeds into my recollections, especially in one particular way: I often *sound* better in my memories than I actually *was*.

I started keeping a journal in the hospital soon after the brain injury. It began as a way to interact with others as I rebuilt my fundamental language skills. But it also became a record of my recovery. Throughout this book, I include journal entries I wrote in the year following the ruptured aneurysm. There were almost no audio or video recordings made of me in my acute stages, so this is likely the closest thing I have to capture my aphasic "voice." Over the span of twelve months, what appeared on the page changed substantially—a portrait of a mind in reconstruction.

In the throes of my recovery, many of my thought patterns felt unfamiliar to me, and since I had been informed early on that I was living with a language disorder, I suspected language was somehow related to this altered cognition. In the years following my injury, and as my ability to read improved, I slowly sought out models about how language and thought intersect, anything that felt especially relevant to my case. I take a multidisciplinary approach in this book. I include a range of resources, from medical to academic, therapeutic to linguistic, and, of course, anything that came from my own personal experience. Questions of how language affects thought have been asked for centuries. Theoretical models and practical research each illuminate the discussion in certain ways, but they also can directly contradict each other. And since these issues remain open-ended in society at large, this book reflects that lack of certainty. Long after my onset of aphasia, I came to know many other people with the condition, and several members of this community reported to me that their experiences with aphasia didn't much resemble my own. I found this difference initially jarring, but soon realized that I shouldn't have been surprised. Language is not one-size-fits-all. Language is unique to each person who uses it, and when it breaks down at a neurological level—like in cases of aphasia—it follows that this experience would also be unique to the individual.

Even though I have regained a lot of my fluency, people with aphasia live with its effects throughout their lifetimes—I certainly do. This does put me in a strange position as the author here. I use language to describe a lack of it, chronicling a journey that troubled my very sense of self, which still makes me wonder what "recovery" can be when considered in such a relative way. After all, what is a memory without a stable identity attached to it? How well could a woman with a language disorder actually recall what people said to her and what she said in response? How could she capture recollections of thought patterns, and how could she come close to relaying how her brain functioned after her brain ceased to function in that way? It is a challenge to say the least, but one propelled by a deep curiosity. Still, with an exploration like this, I think it's only fair to question what is likely to be included and what is bound to be excluded, too. Who would trust that woman with a quotation mark if she could not trust herself?

What I am certain of is this: even though throughout this book I've included journal entries and a few other devices, hoping to accurately represent the way I was thinking during the time of the injury, I also know that some part of this project is impossible because my mind—and my ability to use it—has changed irrevocably since then. And if the person who wrote those journals in 2007–2008 had been able to finish this book at the time, that story wouldn't look or sound anything like this one. I paid attention to the world differently then, and drew different conclusions from what I took in. That's just the kind of paradox I have to know and accept—with no small amount of humor—at every step along the way. "Myself" is a moving target.

AUGUST 23, 2007

The walls of Priscilla's Bar were the color of dark velvet, the wooden floors were sticky, and the air smelled of recently applied cleaning products. The place was far from packed. When my friends and I walked through the front door, we joined a clientele that was middle-aged, disproportionately male and gay. A one-legged man was parked in his wheelchair by the cigarette machine, his large German shepherd panting by his side. He didn't appear to be blind, but the management didn't seem to care about the dog, which I felt added to the genuine come-as-you-are atmosphere of the place. I picked up my drink and headed to a table with my friend Laura. Our other pal, BJ, stayed on at the bar, chatting up the clean-shaven man mixing the drinks. Why pull him away? It was one of our rare nights off from our grueling international tour, and we all needed to unwind in our own way.

We had found the pub during our first week in Scotland, riding buses around town as we prepared our play for its debut at the International Fringe Festival in Edinburgh. Priscilla's was on our bus route, halfway between the theater where we were touring our show and the family home where we were staying. The steep landscapes of Edinburgh were impressive, its parks and graveyards were a verdant patchwork, and the nearby hills were so green they were almost purple. But we soon discovered how much rain was needed to maintain that lushness. Even the sunniest of days would often erupt into spontaneous storms, which swelled the gutters and flooded the routes we would have walked, making our bus commute a necessity. As we sat in our favorite seats at the top level of the red double decker, we would look over at the bar and its patrons, who always started their drinking early. Even the grimmest weather did not dissuade them from squeezing onto the sidewalk in their violet café chairs, cackling over their fluorescent-colored cocktails.

Without a care in the world, Laura would say, leaving her wet fingertips on the fogged-up window as we hurtled by. I understood what she meant. I also had twinges of envy as I looked over that scene. These men were doing exactly what they wanted to do in the exact way they wanted to do it. They seemed so damn satisfied. If only we all could be that lucky.

Laura had written a surreal one-woman play, a tragicomic story of a new-age peace activist with a public access TV show who goes on an ill-conceived hunger strike. The play premiered in a downtown theater in Manhattan with a small but encouraging reception. When it was accepted into the festival in Edinburgh, Laura asked BJ and me to be her touring company. Although we had trained as actors side by side at New York University a decade earlier, we had gathered plenty of experience in the technical and design aspects of theater as well. And we knew we could travel together because we had shared an apartment for a few years. BJ and I accepted Laura's offer without any hesitation, in part because we were happy to help, but mostly because we were looking forward to reliving our days as bunkmates and drinking buddies. But our excitement for our international adventure died down soon after our arrival. The Royal Mile, the main artery of town, was supersaturated with more than three thousand productions, and the city was teeming with bodies, creating a scene that was part Brazilian carnival, part high school pep rally, part mosh pit. As we tried to navigate it all on our first day, I worried about what I had gotten myself into. Though BJ and I knew people who had successfully brought their productions to the Fringe, we hadn't thought to consult with them or get their advice. Between the two of us, we were responsible for everything from costumes and lighting, to sets and promotion. Our lack of organization showed. The second day of the festival didn't improve the situation: after we registered with the Fringe coordinators, we were directed to a back alley, under a bridge, past a Dumpster and a Porta Potty, to a space that looked half abandoned. That was our venue. There had been too many people and too much action on the Mile, but there was definitely not enough of either here. Our new theater wasn't even a theater, but a temporarily repurposed church basement referred to as "The Vault." We were exhausted not only by the demands of our touring schedule but by the mayhem of the festival in this city we barely knew.

When we finally got around to visiting Priscilla's in person, it was a Thursday night, near the end of our tour. It hadn't been the easiest couple of weeks. The number of plays in the festival outstripped the demand from the local audience, so the turnout for most shows was poor. We were finding it impossible to fill our seats, and one night, Laura had to cancel a show entirely because not a single person showed up. All we wanted to do was escape the bleakness of our trip, to disappear for a while, and Priscilla's served this purpose well. On the outskirts of the city, the bar was half empty, and the ubiquitous Fringe guides that were scattered around most of the cafés and pubs around town were noticeably absent on these unwiped tables.

Two tipsy young men were using a column for some amateur pole dancing, though the larger group wasn't paying much attention. A disco ball rotated clunkily overhead, its reflective mosaic lighting up the cracked plaster on the dark walls. Music was emanating from a stage at the back.

As we found seats at a table, a greying man, sturdy as a dockworker, crooned a surprisingly tender karaoke rendition of "Sweet Caroline" into the microphone.

Look sharp, ladies, BJ said as he joined us. He had a drink in one hand and a three-ring binder in the other. That's your competition up there.

What do you mean? I asked. My exhaustion turned to suspicion when I saw the sly grin on BJ's face. What did you do?

Nothing, he said. Nothing bad, anyway. I just signed you and Laura up for the big karaoke contest tonight! He slid the folder of songs across the table and beamed at us.

Come on, Beej, I groaned. I don't want to be stuck in here all night.

Lauren, I know this festival has been more like a stress-tival until now, but need I remind you of the extensive performance training shared among the three of us? Are you honestly saying you don't think that you and Laura can take the title of the best karaoke duet of the night? Or is there another bee in your bonnet? He shimmied up next to me. Because you know what I think? I think you're just upset you can't get your flirt on here. . . .

I swatted at BJ playfully. A Scottish romance had definitely not been in my plan for this trip; I had someone back home. Sort of. My boyfriend, Jonah, and I had been on and off for five years, and though our relationship was complicated, it was far from over. But a harmless tête-à-tête with a handsome stranger would have been a welcome distraction, and there was absolutely no way that was going to happen here.

Come on, Lauren, BJ said. Pleeeease.

BJ was being a little pushy, but I knew he simply wanted to make the most of this trip. He had left NY for a while, and after spending some time in the Peace Corps, the Fringe was his return to theater life. And he had recently been admitted into a post-baccalaureate program at Columbia University, now on the path to becoming a medical doctor. Nights out like this would be a rare occurrence once we got home. And I had to consider Laura, too. The show's lack of traction, reviews, and audience had been hard for me and BJ to face, but Laura was the writer and sole performer, and she was bearing the brunt of the failure. Now, as she flipped through the song listings, I noticed that she was smiling for the first time in weeks.

There's got to be some prize money for the winner, Laura said. Or at least free drinks.

BJ nudged me affectionately. Go tread the boards a bit. I bet it will make you feel better, he said.

I didn't give BJ the satisfaction of agreeing with him aloud, but he was probably right—in spite of my protestations otherwise, getting onstage almost always improved my mood. Raised by two former actors in Los Angeles, I had been performing before I had gotten out of diapers. Even if I was tired, even if it was a silly duet in a sparsely populated dive bar, this kind of self-expression both enlivened and relaxed me.

Laura had been hoping to come to Priscilla's since she first laid eyes on it, and I was already talking about leaving. That was just bad form. Of course I could stay a little longer. If I still wanted to explore the town later, I could sneak away afterward. I would set out on my own.

Well? BJ asked me.

I stuck my tongue out at him, but then I let him choose our song.

When the bartender-emcee called out our names, BJ quickly set the video function on his camera to record, and Laura and I climbed onstage. The synthesized track cued up to "Total Eclipse of the Heart." We put our arms around each other's shoulders as the white lyrics on the screen turned to yellow, and we started the song.

I don't remember when I stopped singing. I don't remember the fall.

It was a slap that roused me. I wasn't awake yet, not really, because even then my eyelids refused to open. Was that a slap across my face? Even in that drowsy haze, I knew that the world of bodies had changed. Fingertips, skin, groin; all had a new viscous life. Everything was in the wrong place. I was certain it was a dream; it could only be a dream, and I wished my mother would wake me up.

Then, another slap.

As my eyes began to focus, it wasn't my mother I saw hovering above me, but a man identifying himself as a medic. He became broader and blurrier as I was lifted from the bar floor. He was talking to me but I couldn't understand him exactly. My ears weren't on right. It felt important to let him know that I wasn't drunk. But my mouth wasn't on right either. My gaze narrowed for a moment, down toward my legs. One foot was still strapped into my high, black heels, but the other foot was wriggling and naked, and then, everything in my field of vision started to wobble toward darkness. Voices I didn't know and hands I didn't recognize slid me onto a stretcher. An ambulance door slammed shut, I vomited into a canister someone handed to me, and the warping howl of a Scottish siren began to echo between my ears. I was out of breath and my eyes were tearing. I felt something like panic, and then not. I felt something like pain, and then not. I started to drown.

PART ONE

THE QUIET

*Aphasia, the loss of language following brain injury,
is devastating, and in severe cases family members
may feel that the whole person is lost forever.*
STEVEN PINKER, *The Language Instinct*

1

In my memories of the Scottish hospital, the sky is always blue, though I know that can't be completely accurate. Summer was waning, and as my friends and I had already experienced, Edinburgh was prone to unpredictable storms. Yet, I can't think of a single moment of rain in the two weeks I lay in bed. My morphine-soaked haze only allowed glimpses and fragments: the bracing air coming in from an open window, the rough comfort of my mother's fingers wiping my fever-moist brow, my father's tears. All of that must have been confusing to me, but when I think of this time, I remember more clarity than confusion. I remember the Quiet.

This was not a Quiet I had known before. It was a placid current, a presence more than an absence. Everything I saw or touched or heard pulsed with a marvelous sense of order. I had a nothing mind, a flotsam mind. I was incredibly focused on the present, with very little awareness or interest in my past or future. My entire environment felt interconnected, like cells in a large, breathing organism. To experience this Quiet was to be it.

However, this sense of serenity was not shared by those around me.

After the medics had taken me away in an ambulance, Laura and BJ had called my parents in the US. It was the middle of the night in Edinburgh, but early evening in Los Angeles, and no one was overly worried about my fall from the stage, since it appeared I was suffering a simple concussion. That all changed two hours after my hospital admission—when the results of my CT scan showed the actual crisis unfolding. An aneurysm had ruptured in my brain and the hemorrhage was spreading. A neuroradiologist explained to my parents how precarious my situation was—how often people died the instant an aneurysm ruptured, and even after treatment, only slightly more than half of these patients actually survive the next few days. With every second being critical, the doctor was preparing for an emergency operation. But my now-horrified parents were stranded in California. Their passports were in their safety deposit box, and the bank branch was closed for the night. My parents rattled on the windows of the bank the next morning, successfully convincing them to open early for them because there was no time to waste. My procedure was well under way when my parents boarded their flight the next morning, leaving my brother and grandmother behind at the house. The operation was already over when they got to Edinburgh. My parents and friends came together, relieved that I had survived the operation, but living with a keen awareness of how perilous my situation still was.

It took a few days for me to wake up fully, under the influence of a combination of swollen brain tissue and heavy sedation. However, when I was more alert, the Quiet I found myself experiencing was much more interesting than my medical state. I had woken up to a new world, hushed, and full of curiosities.

One of these moments of marvel took place during a move between the critical unit and the recovery ward. I was being transported in a mirrored elevator, and although there were no bandages on my face and my vision was clear, it was almost impossible for me to recognize my own reflection. Yet, somehow, this didn't disturb me. In fact, it made remarkable sense because I was quickly realizing that my reflection was not the only thing that was different. Transformation felt abundant. Once-fixed concepts, like "wall" and "window," weren't as easy to identify anymore, and the differences between "he" and "she" and "I" and "it" were becoming indistinguishable. I knew my parents were my parents and my friends were my friends, but I felt less like myself and more like everything around me.

I was wheeled to a bed by a westerly-facing window, with three other women in the room. My suitemates were often in discussion with one another. Even through their brogues, I understood what they were saying, but I rarely took part in the conversations. I just enjoyed the way their voices plodded and pattered like footsteps.

At this point I didn't know much about my brain injury at all. I wasn't in any pain, so my thoughts about my new condition were unfocused and fleeting. Instead of being occupied by questions about why I was in the hospital and what had happened to me, my mind was engrossed in an entirely different set of perceptions. The smallest of activities would enthrall me. Dressing myself, I was awed by the orbital distance between cloth and flesh. Brushing my teeth, I was enchanted by the stiffness of the bristles and the sponginess of my gums. I also spent an inordinate amount of time looking out the window. My view was mainly of the hospital's rooftop, with its grey and untextured panels, though I developed a lot of interest in a nearby tree. I could only make out the tops of the branches, but I'd watch this section of needles and boughs intently, fascinated by how the slightest wind would change the shape entirely. It was always and never the same tree.

Very few things disturbed me during this period of time. But even in this formless daydream I remember the moment that most closely resembled real distress. Or, at least, when I became aware of an actual loss.

It must have been midday because the sunlight was falling across my body, and that slat of light emphasized the white nightstand on my left. My parents had filled the shelves inside with clothing, and the nurses made sure there were plenty of liquids for me to drink in there, too. On this day, I noticed that there was a stack of magazines on the nightstand, as well as a book. I am not sure how long they had been there—for all I knew, they could have even predated my arrival—but this was the first time they piqued my interest.

The high gloss of the magazine cover felt wet in my hands. And as I opened it up, I was instantly bombarded with photos of red carpet parades and illustrated makeup tips, a circus of color and distraction. I couldn't linger anywhere. It felt as if the magazine were shouting at me. Closing it was a relief.

I turned to the book. It was a novel by Agatha Christie, something I had probably read many years earlier. I opened to chapter one and flipped slowly and evenly through the first few pages, a motion that seemed to come naturally to me. But on the third page, I stopped. I returned to the first page and started again. Slower this time. Much slower. My eyes focused and refocused in the bright sunlight, but I continued to only see the black, blocked shapes where words used to be.

Thinking about it now, I don't know how I could be so certain that it was an Agatha Christie novel, especially since this was the very moment I became aware I couldn't read anymore. With this simultaneously familiar and unfamiliar book in my hands, I first took in the actual loss of words. For my entire life, language had been at the forefront of every personal or professional achievement, and very few things had brought me as much joy and purpose. If I had ever been warned that I might be robbed of my ability to read, even for a limited amount of time, it would have been a devastation too cruel to bear. Or so I would have thought. But a day did come when I couldn't read the book in front of me, when paragraphs appeared to be nothing more than senseless jumbles, and the way I actually processed this massive loss was surprisingly mild. The knowledge of the failure was jarring, without a doubt, but was there any misery or angst? No. My reaction was much less sharp. A vague sense of disappointment swept through me, but then . . . my inability to use words in this way just felt like transient information. Now that the ability was gone, I could no longer think of how or why it should have any influence on my life whatsoever.

It's shocking to reflect on that moment, and think about how the loss of something so crucial washed past me with such a vague wisp of emotion. But I was living so deeply in the present—and in the comfort of the Quiet—I couldn't fully realize how my sense of identity had shifted. It would be several weeks before I detected how much of myself had gone missing, and how hard I'd have to fight to regain it. However, the unpleasant sensations that came with holding that book drifted away as soon as I closed it. And with no effort at all, my attention settled back on the impossible blue sky.

2

A few days after the surgery and a battery of tests, Dr. Rustam Al-Shahi Salman, the consultant neurologist overseeing my case, made my parents aware of the short- and long-term issues at hand. Dr. Salman was slim and soft-spoken, his gestures and words thoughtful, and he was never rushed, a demeanor that fit nicely in the Quiet I now inhabited. He was also probably the first person who used the word *aphasia* with my family. However, he explained it in much more detail with my parents than with me.

He told my parents that aphasia did not attack a person's cognitive abilities and most often left a person's intelligence completely intact. But this condition could manifest quite differently in different people, and aphasia is generally divided into two categories: *receptive* and *expressive*. Expressive aphasia (also called "non-fluent" or "Broca's" aphasia) is characterized by word-finding difficulties, while receptive aphasia (also called "fluent" or "Wernicke's" aphasia) affects language comprehension. The expressive issues were most pronounced in my case, but in the beginning, I struggled with receptive issues, too, unable to detect the missing or garbled parts of my own language.

The speech and language therapist Dr. Salman appointed to me aimed to change that.

Anne Rowe was near my mother's age, with faded red curls cut close to her head. For a while, it seemed to me that her only job was to hand me worksheets. Piles and piles of worksheets. One of the first worksheets she gave me had a panel of faces. Every day I was instructed to point at the bald man in the images to tell her how I was feeling.

I feel fine, I said. Or thought I said. But Anne would insist on a more in-depth answer.

Why don't you just try to point to the picture that feels most appropriate for you? she would ask.

It didn't occur to me then that Anne was employing this image prompt not as an exercise but a necessity—because most of the time she couldn't understand my responses to her questions. While my expressive aphasia prevented me from speaking clearly, my receptive aphasia prevented me from knowing when my language was not clear. According to my parents, in the first two weeks I could only say forty or fifty words.

Anne's records from our initial sessions mention that creating the sounds for speech was often challenging for me too: "Lauren is able to use fully intact phrases at times without hesitation, but has clear difficulties with word finding and motor planning for speech." This meant I had trouble shaping my mouth to make the right sounds—a condition known as *speech apraxia*, which often accompanies an onset of aphasia. Children go through a similar process, stuttering into speech while parents ask them to repeat and refine what they are saying until they do it correctly. Anne's worksheets had the same goal. Pointing at a drawing of a mouth, she'd say: The tip of the tongue goes here. . . .

Then she would illustrate on her own face: T, T, T, Teh, is the tip of the tongue. Th, Th, Th is Thuh, the fat part of the tongue.

I wasn't disturbed when Anne asked me to take part in these articulation exercises. They didn't indicate to me that there was something especially wrong. In fact, they strongly resembled the routine vocal warm-ups

I had been doing—and enjoying—since theater school. Asking an actor to demonstrate the difference between a *P* sound and a *B* sound over and over was nothing out of the ordinary. When I was instructed to do so in the hospital, I assumed I was excelling at it, flexing my muscle memory, until Anne subtly indicated my failures and misfires with her feedback throughout our sessions.

Very good, she'd say. Or: not exactly, try again.

At some point, I realized that Anne was saying "not exactly" a lot. And if we hit too many "try agains", Anne would suggest we move on to something else for a while. It was a major hint that something was amiss. I didn't know exactly what was wrong, but I would try to fix it because I preferred positive feedback to negative.

One week after the rupture, Anne administered the Western Aphasia Battery test on me. After the reading section, she made this note: "Testing was stopped as Lauren was becoming distressed. L. is very aware she could not do task." Though I have a hard time remembering this distress, I trust in Anne's reporting. My best guess is that my anxiety was only skin deep and short-lived. I also believe my awareness was more limited than Anne might have assumed. I probably wasn't thinking about my inability to do this task and how that might affect my limitations on future tasks. At the time, I had very little concern for the past or future; but in the present, I simply didn't like to disappoint. That, more than anything, was probably the source of my distress. Lucky for me, though, it didn't last long. In the way I perceived the world, negative impressions could pass very quickly, as if I had never even had them.

My trouble with spoken language was mirrored in my written language. I discovered as I progressed in my sessions with Anne that I had not completely forgotten the alphabet, but I had forgotten its order. If I isolated single letters at a time, I could still identify them on a page. It took a lot of guidance from Anne, but with her by my side, I could slowly sound out these letters, occasionally creating a very fragile word. Anne noted: "There are frequent errors reading aloud, especially words with irregular pronunciations, and Lauren finds it difficult to know if she is correct or not." So, while I had not lost my ability to read entirely, "reading" in this new iteration of my life involved a razor-sharp focus, accommodating only a word at a time. I also wasn't able to know my own accuracy without someone else's support. I would slowly sound out a word, but it took so long that when I went on to tackle the next one, I often would forget what I had just read. Perhaps that was what had happened with the "Agatha Christie" book I had attempted to read by myself. I had been expecting the language on the page to behave the way it used to, and when it didn't, the whole picture crumbled in front of me. Words could be approachable in small, isolated units. But a full sentence? That was beyond imagining.

Aphasia can affect a patient's hearing, too. Though Anne was quick to confirm that this was not an issue in my case, she mentioned in her notes that I needed a fair amount of repetition. My parents also noticed that I sometimes asked them to repeat themselves, but this was much more common between Anne and me. I was an American being instructed by a Scottish speech therapist on how to use the English language. Anne used a slightly different inflection on her words, and that sometimes made her speech radically strange to me. These occasionally ridiculous elements of our interactions were just par for the course. This was when my language was at its most vulnerable. She just didn't identify the world in the ways my parents or friends did. Plenty of things got lost in translation. What she called a *cushion*, my mother would call a *pillow*; what she called a *loo*, my father would call a *bathroom*. And whenever the topic of lunch came up, we couldn't always sort out the menu because the way she said *herb* or *tomato* hit all the wrong chords in me.

But Anne was a consummate professional. I realize now that Anne was trying to address a systematic failure in me: my newly acquired aphasia. I just couldn't think of it like that. I could flip-flop in our exchanges and not hear the mistakes. When I did, I would assume I was simply tired or that the disturbances were all minor and temporary. And as soon as our session would end, I would gently be redelivered to the happy stillness of the pervasive Quiet.

Language was something I had never struggled with before, so it was hard to believe it could be a problem now. I don't know if Anne could appreciate this blissful ignorance in me, but she was experienced and practical enough to know that any of my next steps could not be taken alone. All of her reports emphasized that I was still in the acute stages and that everyone close to me was going to be as involved in this process as I was.

3

When my parents had arrived from California, they joined Laura and BJ in Edinburgh, staying in a local family's home. The Patersons were friends of friends, and they had allowed us to lodge with them during our Fringe tour, free of charge. When our trip took this much more serious turn, Alan and Alison Paterson welcomed my parents just as warmly as they had welcomed BJ, Laura, and me. My parents and friends had known one another for years, and since they were now all living under the same roof, they usually visited me in the hospital en masse.

In these early weeks post rupture, I had a very shaky sense of personal recollection, lacking all sorts of details from my own life, but I wasn't suffering from amnesia. I knew truth from fiction. And even though I had trouble saying or writing the names of the people around me, I certainly knew who they were and what sort of role they played in my life.

Explicit memories, also called *autobiographic* memories, are the ones we can call up in the form of conscious recall, often things that have made a strong emotional impact on us. *Implicit* memories are subtler than that, usually procedural in nature—things that may have shaped our abilities and talents long ago and continue to inform our current decisions at the unconscious level. We don't know why some memories are forgotten and others persist like wounds that never close. But while my explicit memories floundered, my implicit memories, like how to bring a straw to my lips, were completely retained. Memories don't exist in a single location, so encoding or retrieving them activates many parts of your brain. And actually, the company we keep can also affect the way in which we recall autobiographical memory. Though I was mentally rooted in the present, my friends and family often wanted to talk about the past. When coaxed by them, I could slowly recall people, places, or events, though when I did, these memories simply didn't bring strong sensations with them. This frustrated the people around me. They wanted me to feel the way I always felt, enjoy the things I used to enjoy. But it wasn't that simple for me.

One afternoon in early September, this large group arrived for visiting hours. After giving me a long, lingering hug, my parents stood together by the rocking chair while BJ perched on the wide windowsill. Laura planted herself on the corner of my inclined bed, took off her oversize brown windbreaker, and twisted her long hair up into a bun.

She took out a piece of paper that had a sort of collage of dozens of thumb-size images.

Let's start in the lower left hand corner of this page, Laura said. Because this image is probably the hardest one to recognize. That's the gag gift you gave BJ a few years ago: Billy the Big Mouthed Bass. Do you see how the fish is *singing*? The way you liked to sing . . .

I looked at this photo of a plastic fish—a little nonplussed. Apparently I liked to sing.

What about this? Laura was pointing at one of her thumb-size pictures again. *Kale*, she said. Remember how you like to prepare kale with sesame seeds?

I looked at the rendering of the bumpy, dark vegetable. Okay, I liked kale. That seemed possible, though it didn't seem especially relevant at the moment.

Laura continued, undeterred. There was a picture of a football stadium, and Laura pointed at that, too. It's the Rose Bowl, she said. It's in Pasadena, California. Your family lives in Pasadena.

Altadena, actually, my dad corrected her. That's where the house is, but our office is in Pasadena. It's the *Pasadena* in *Pasadena Advertising*. And Lauren knows that one, don't you, kiddo? Because that's the company your mom and I set up when you kids were little.

Now, my mother took her turn speaking to me. Mike has been missing you terribly, and he really wanted to be here, she said. I am sure you've been wondering why we left your little brother behind. . . .

In fact, I hadn't been wondering that at all. Not until my mother mentioned it, at least. My brother and I were the only children in this family. Almost seven years apart, I had been one of his main caregivers as a child, and we had remained close as adults. Now a sophomore in college in Northern California, he would call me with some regularity in New York. We'd catch up or talk about a movie we'd both seen, or he'd need advice about something he didn't want to ask our folks about. But if my mother hadn't mentioned him, I might even have forgotten I had a brother.

That kind of extreme forgetfulness seems so incongruous to me now, so impossible, but this was just the kind of disruption I was experiencing within my autobiographic memories. Previously, like most neurotypical people, at a moment's notice a certain word, sound, or smell could transport me out of my current time and place; thousands of invisible strands would be plucked simultaneously, cross-referencing a lifetime of experiences, weaving together a rapid emotional tapestry, and producing a complex feeling. But my thoughts in the hospital rarely made this mental time travel. Instead, I could only focus on what was directly in front of me. Right here. Right now.

I often wonder how much my aphasic language played a role in this disjointed memory retrieval process. Words had always been powerful triggers for me, capable of bringing forth evocative memories, but they didn't have that same potency anymore. Everyone who came to these visiting-hours sessions has told me that I gestured and nodded and seemed to understand what people were saying, but I didn't contribute to the conversations much.

My sentences were short, and my grammar was shot. From my decimated vocabulary, I could only put together two or three words in a row. My father says he did (somewhat) enjoy the sort of words I unwittingly coined back then (like *emborrosing*—when I combined the words *boring* and *embarrassing*), and he also says I cursed and slurred like a drunken sailor. My mother tells me I said the word *time* a lot. *Time* this and *time* that, *time* when it didn't make any sense in the context at all. And, of course, I didn't hear any of these problems myself.

Laura returned to her images for a final push. She pointed at a new picture, this one taken near my current apartment.

Greenpoint, Lauren. You live in Greenpoint, Brooklyn.

Her finger pushed to an image of a school crest.

You're in *grad school*, pursuing a PhD in theater.

She directed me to a photo of men in ties, standing in line.

You just received a *teaching fellowship* from Baruch College.

With little response from me, BJ unraveled his tangle of limbs from the windowsill and stretched his long legs to the floor. What about the play, Lauren? Can you remember the show we brought from New York to the Fringe? And the whole stress-tival?

He turned to Laura. Maybe we should remind her of some of the productions we saw during the Fringe? But then again, maybe we're doing her a disservice. Most of those plays were so miserable they weren't worthy of anyone's attention, let alone a commemoration.

My father guffawed at BJ's snark. My parents, former actors themselves, found his low-level gossipmongering a guilty pleasure, and soon their voices became a chattering knot. I liked that my family and friends enjoyed one another, but when there were too many sounds in a room, it all started to blur together. They were discussing recent events, but since I didn't feel connected to those events anymore, I started to tune out the conversation entirely.

Laura noticed and leaned over the bed, hoping to recapture my attention.

Do you remember the bar, Lauren? You and I singing in Priscilla's Bar?

Was I meant to say something? Do something? My confusion was now teetering on all-out frustration. What did Laura need from me? Want from me? At least soft-spoken Anne was slower on her worksheets and gave me time to think.

I realize now that my friends and family were simply trying to be proactive on my behalf. They had been told that a feeling might incite a bit of language, or some language might incite a feeling. But this just wasn't happening that afternoon. The only reason I took part in these exercises wasn't because the material mattered to me, but because it seemed to matter to everyone else.

My life had always been populated with big personalities, and I had created different approaches as a way to interact with each of them—as a daughter, as an older sister, as an actress, as a roommate, as a girlfriend. Before the stroke, my ability to appreciate the needs and desires of these complex characters around me came pretty easily. But after the stroke, my emotional sensitivity had dulled tremendously. It was hard to know what other people might be thinking, and I wasn't that interested in finding out. My general disinterest in interpersonal interactions was probably rooted in both emotional and anatomical aspects.

The rupture had originated on the middle cerebral artery in the left hemisphere of my brain, bleeding into the Sylvian fissures and my left basal ganglia. This cerebral artery supplies the blood for the two language centers of the brain—Broca's Area and Wernicke's Area. The basal ganglia are usually associated with motor control, but they also affect habits, cognition, and emotion. Some basal injuries can blunt emotional awareness and slow "goal-directed" activity. With such a wide range of influences, the alterations to the basal ganglia were probably affecting me in many ways at the time, but after the rupture, it was my faltering language that was my most visible symptom.

My aphasia had invisible effects, too, in ways that many people wouldn't even think about. It was not just my external language that was ailing. My inner monologue, my self-directed speech, had also gone almost completely mute. In its place was the radiant Quiet. The nourishing Quiet. The illuminating Quiet.

The Quiet was not something I spoke to anyone about. While my parents were on alert for signs of a secondary stroke (*vasospasms* are common after a rupture), I was happy enough floating in this meditative state. It felt deeply unique to me, but I later learned of other people (who also sustained damage to the left hemisphere of the brain) who have reported similar phenomena. Clinical psychologist Scott Moss describes waking up in the hospital with his own aphasia. His account is included in *Injured Brains of Medical Minds*. He writes:

> "I did comprehend somewhat vaguely what was said to me. . . . I
> didn't have any difficulty focusing: it was simply that the words,
> individually or in combination, didn't have meaning, and even more
> amazing, I was only a trifle bothered by that. . . . I had also lost the
> ability even to engage in self-talk. . . . I simply existed. . . . It was as if
> without words I could not be concerned about tomorrow."

And Jill Bolte Taylor, a Harvard-trained neuroanatomist, who is well-known for being the author of the bestseller *My Stroke of Insight*, lost this inner monologue as well. She describes it as "brain chatter" that was "replaced by a pervasive and enticing inner peace." In addition, she writes that she "didn't think in the same way," partially because of the "dramatic silence that had taken residency" in her. Bolte Taylor specifically identifies her perceptual changes as related to a shift of attention between the two hemispheres of her brain.

In *The Master and His Emissary: The Divided Brain and the Making of the Western World*, psychiatrist and writer Iain McGilchrist goes much further into detail about the differences between these hemispheres. The brain looks like a walnut split down the middle, and its two lobes are called *hemispheres*. Each is a fully functional processing unit, like a PC and Mac side by side in the skull. Though they usually work together to create a seemingly uniform worldview, a human being can live with only one functional hemisphere, or one hemisphere can do the heavy lifting while the other is under repair (as is often the case for a person who has suffered a stroke). McGilchrist takes issue with the pseudoscience of people calling themselves "left-brained" or "right-brained," but that being said, the hemispheres do have different strengths, or as McGilchrist describes it, their differences deal with "competing needs" and "the types of attention they are required to bring to bear on the world." This bifurcated arrangement doesn't just exist in humans, but in most vertebrates, too. In a single moment, a bird, using its left hemisphere, must identify if an item is food or sand and using its right hemisphere, simultaneously be on guard for predators. McGilchrist mentions that these are "two quite different kinds of exercise, requiring not just that attention should be divided, but that it should be two distinct types (of attention) at once."

These hemispheric differences are not so divergent in humans, only more sophisticated. Our left hemisphere is much more detail-focused, and since both language centers exist on this side of the brain, it is much more verbal. But the right hemisphere has a keen awareness, too, and it is more vigilant than the left, more receptive to new information. McGilchrist writes:

"The left hemisphere's 'stickiness,' its tendency to recur to what it is
familiar with, tends to reinforce whatever it is already doing. There
is a reflexivity to the process, as if trapped in a hall of mirrors: it only
discovers more of what it already knows, and it only does more of
what it already is doing. The right hemisphere by contrast (is) seeing
more of the picture, and taking a broader perspective."

This description resonates intensely with me. Without language, I was paying attention to the world in a new way. Without the talents and abilities I had once relied on—and used to identify myself—I was interacting with more ineffable senses. I had escaped from my old hall of mirrors, and with my language-dominant left hemisphere somewhat disabled, I was probably taking in a whole host of perceptions from the right hemisphere that were suddenly prioritized.

I was experiencing a near-constant sensation of interconnectedness, but my observations often lacked specific categories and dimensions, and a sense of my own personal preference. My "self" didn't seem at all pertinent in this kind of processing. It was all happening to me and through me, but not necessarily because of me.

I believe this temporary shift—changing the dominance from one hemisphere to the other and losing my inner voice for a while—was a huge part of what made the Quiet so quiet. The constant stream of language, which I had always assumed was thought, had stopped. It's hard to describe this voice exactly, and even harder to describe its lack. It is the internal monologue that turns on in the morning, when we instruct ourselves to "Get up" and "Make breakfast." It's a voice we use to monitor ourselves, to criticize or to doubt—and it can be pernicious this way. However, it can be an effective tool as well. We can motivate ourselves with it, understand our environment better, and sometimes modify our situations as well. My inner speech returned very slowly, not on a certain day, but in bits and bobs. In the hospital, though, I didn't realize that I no longer had access to it, only that something in me felt substantially . . . different.

However, I certainly was able to think after the aneurysm's rupture. In many ways, my thinking had never been clearer. I retained the capacity for complex thought, but it was not represented by words or phrases, and my ideas didn't cluster or activate one another the same way. It wasn't ignorance, but there was an element of innocence.

And on the whole, this silence served me very well. With my internal monologue on mute, I was mainly spared from understanding my condition early on. Unable to ask myself: *What is wrong with me?* I could not, and did not, list the many things that were.

I was no longer the narrator of my own life.

When you don't have words to probe and investigate the world, mystery can exist everywhere. My own body was a landscape of enigmas. For instance,

I could still use my right arm, my dominant arm, and feel pressure there during my neurological exams. But it felt light, almost hollow.

And there was my head, too. Doctors and family members had told me that I was a brain patient, yet I had walked my fingers around my head and I hadn't found a scar or even a bump there. So how could I have undergone brain surgery? The only part of my body that was sore was my upper leg, and that hardly seemed related to my brain.

Later, I learned that a stroke to the left hemisphere of the brain affects the motor skills on the right side of the body. That was why I had that hollow, doll-like feeling in my hand.

As for my head? My doctors hadn't gone through the skull at all during my operation. It was a neuroradiological procedure. An incision had been made near my groin, where the doctors accessed the femoral artery. A neuroradiologist had pushed a thin wire and a camera up a surgical catheter through the length of my body. When it arrived in my brain, the camera oversaw the work as the wire was compacted into tight coils, blocking the aneurysm from the rest of the blood flow. That explained the discomfort in my groin.

When people ask me these days, I describe the procedure a bit like putting a cork in a bottle of wine. But closer to the time of the actual experience, any descriptions at all would have felt irrelevant. My arm was just my arm. My head was just my head. Both were the same, and not at all the same, as they had always been.

And such were the little mysteries I could live inside of.

4

My parents and I have very different memories of the day I drew them a map in the hospital. They remember this being one of my most difficult periods of time, after the rupture itself. And I remember it as the day I drank the World's Best Diet Pepsi. But all of us agree this was a turning point, a moment in which I became more active in my own recovery.

The morning started out in the best possible way. One of my suitemates had told me she wanted to go down to the vending machines on the ground floor of the hospital and invited me to join her. It was a thrilling proposition, since I had never ventured past the recovery ward. My bare feet welcomed the coolness of the stone steps and linoleum underfoot. I had no money on me, didn't even think of it before we arrived at our destination, but my suitemate was more than happy to buy me a soda. The volcanic sweetness fizzed across my lips, and a kind of raucous joy sparkled across my tongue. Though I had certainly drunk sodas in the past, the entire sensation felt explosively new.

We returned upstairs, and my parents arrived as I was finishing the final drops of my soda. I tried to tell them about this incredible sensation still lingering in my mouth, but the more I tried to express my cheer, the more concerned they seemed to become. To them, I was speaking almost exclusively in nonsense, and worse yet, I was completely oblivious to it.

They called Dr. Salman and went to talk to him in the hallway privately, to express their building concern out of my earshot. They told him my language seemed much worse than the day before. He explained that backslides did happen in cases like mine, and the regression might only be temporary. When my parents returned to the room, they came back talking about how I might need more support than they had originally thought. They might need some help. And this was when I said one of my first intelligible words of the day. It was a name, actually: Betsy.

Betsy who? my mom asked. Betsy from high school? Both of my parents were confused. Betsy and I hadn't spoken for years.

I couldn't understand why my mother couldn't understand me. So, I started to draw her a map. I sketched a house in the hills to represent my parents' home in Altadena. Betsy, I said. I traced an intersection at Lake Avenue and Altadena Drive. Betsy, I said again as I pointed. I marked a building at the end of the long line. Betsy. I tapped the destination. Betsy, *Betsy*!

The map itself had only a small relationship to my old friend. I wasn't trying to contact her, but instead was drawing a route to her alma mater, California Institute of Technology. I had no idea if that university treated issues like mine, or even what my issue was exactly. But clearly there was a problem, and some part of me remembered that Caltech was a place where problems were solved.

My parents eventually understood somehow, and when my mother tried contacting Betsy, something incredible—and peculiar—happened. It turned out that her father was the head of the Department of Communication Disorders at a neighboring university, a fact I was completely oblivious to. And, with a position like that, there were very few people in California who knew more about aphasia than he did. He became an invaluable resource for my parents, familiarizing them with the disorder, informing them about what could happen in acute stages, and giving them treatment advice. This was something they desperately needed and his expertise made their next steps navigable.

Afterward, everyone was impressed I had orchestrated this complicated course of action, brought all of these disparate parties together, and even with my limited language skills, sought out the perfect expert for this exact situation. The truth was a little more complicated. In point of fact, I had initially tried to lead my parents in an entirely different direction, but the outcome couldn't have gone any better. It was my first lesson in how there can be a very thin line dividing the mistaken and the miraculous. There can be direction, even in the misstep.

5

Close to three weeks after I had failed to read the book by my bedside, I wandered into the visitors' room at the end of the hall, and resting on the round wooden table was another book. Aside from the strained moments of conversation with other people, which would exacerbate my language loss, I didn't think about it much. I am not sure if I missed reading exactly, I'm not even sure I was capable of that nostalgia or wistfulness, but something about books still drew me in. Even if I couldn't read them, touching them still provided a type of satisfaction. I could enjoy their weight, savor the smell of ink and mildew, and welcome the rough flip of the pages running across my numb right hand.

With my uneven grasp, I picked up the book before me. It was a hardback, and on its cover was an illustration of a man, a cluster of clouds, and a flock of birds. The background was off-white, and the birds were multicolored. The man himself was in silhouette. He stood as if he had just taken a large step forward, with one straight leg in front of the other. He had a telescope to his eye, and he was looking into the distance. I started to thumb through the pages, but as I did so, they assembled into an unexpected kind of order. They shifted and squirmed, and then these patterns suddenly looked a lot like . . . something. These letters looked like words.

But was I actually reading this? Was that even possible? Should I tell someone?

My fingers swept over the bubble of raised ink on the cover, where the book gave me a more formal announcement, calling itself *Cloud of Sparrows*.

It was hard for me to understand what was happening in that moment. Reading, as I had come to experience it recently, always involved Anne. She would point to letters and I would sound them out to her. But I couldn't corral them by myself. With the first book I encountered, which may or may not have been written by Agatha Christie, I'd never know if I had actually been able to read the name of the author, or if I had just recognized aspects of the book as an object—impressions that could have been carried over from my life before. But this new book was different. I had never read it or even seen it until that very moment. I was experiencing everything about it for the very first time.

Cloud. Of. Sparrows. All of these words made sense to me. I knew what a cloud was—I could see them out of my window. I knew a sparrow was an animal and I could call up that image in my mind's eye. Still, I felt I couldn't trust this initial impression. When I actually opened the book, the words inside were too tightly packed, like a net of just-caught fish. So I tried to pluck out individual words at a time. I thought I identified the word *Japan. Japan.* I knew Japan. I had been to Japan. This story might have something to do with Japan. I clutched the book to my breast, pressing it against my quickening heartbeat. I was caught up in a new stream of desire. Now that I had been given a glimpse of what it was like to read, I was overjoyed by the possibility. I just wasn't sure if I was reading yet.

When Anne arrived for our next session, she launched into the day's instruction as usual. I startled her when I reached out and clutched her tiny wrist.

This is important, I tried to say, gesturing to the book. *I think I can read this.*

But saying this aloud felt too bold. Risky somehow. What if Anne proved me wrong?

Anne seemed to understand what I was saying and grabbed a nearby magazine.

Why don't you try to read these sentences? she asked. Take your time.

She came to my side of the bed, silently reading the piece herself, and making notes. It was very slowgoing, but when I said I was done, she gave me her piece of paper and asked her questions aloud, too.

Was this paragraph about A) Europe, B) China, C) Antarctica, or D) the Caribbean?

I pointed and tried to say *Caribbean*.

She nodded and continued. Does the author invite the readers to travel by A) plane, B) boat, C) train, or D) on foot?

I circled *boat* and tried to say it, though I probably stumbled on the diphthong.

Good, Anne said. That's very good.

Though this breakthrough was significant to me, it wasn't particularly life changing, not immediately. My world was still mainly Quiet. And being able to read this little bit of text didn't change my focus on everything. I didn't become hyper-aware of all the written words around me, on signs or in lists. It was still difficult to decipher a lot. I didn't even try to read any more of *Cloud of Sparrows*. Still, it sparked something in me. I immediately identified this as the day I learned to read.

Anne, however, knew we still had a long way to go. Her most pressing objective was to establish my baseline communication. To her, I was in the middle of a complex language re-immersion. She probably wouldn't make blunt distinctions like "the days I couldn't read" and "the day I could." Moments of *spontaneous recovery* like this tend to happen in the first days, or weeks, after an onset of aphasia. The neural mechanisms in this kind of recovery are not well understood, and they manifest dramatically differently from person to person. Some linguistic abilities simply return, other things need to be entirely relearned, and certain capacities can never be fully accessed again.

My reading was important, yes, but much more important was my ability to articulate my needs to others. Speaking, reading, and writing all reinforced each other. Anne told me that when one aspect of language failed, I should just try another approach. When you can't speak, write, she said.

And that was what I started to do. My parents picked up on this quickly and soon bought me my first journal.

Though I can identify "The Day I Learned to Read Again," I can't pinpoint the day I learned to write. It feels like a more nuanced distinction. Anne had given me an alphabet sheet, and I could write words that she had me copy like a four-year-old with a piece of tracing paper. With some cajoling, I did that early, probably in the first week, but my initial journal was a strange primer. It wasn't like the *A is for Apple, O is for Octopus* workbooks I filled in as a kindergartener. It's chock-full of very specific items that represent a very particular life. I could congratulate myself on having pretty good spelling and steady-enough handwriting at the time, but these are somewhat different cognitive processes.

In a few weeks this confetti of fractured words would give way to fractured sentences, too. There was so much I couldn't remember, but having the paper in front of me helped.

When I consider the journals now, I have to read, remember, and imagine.

I imagine. I remember. I translate.

paris museum
paint
weapons
people   6
[art]   lady
    museum
    jeweller
    saint c~~happ~~
        chappele

sun log avro
/lady Cota

mines
bullets
cemetr amor
        ana

tumor

tumor

discovery
channel

specialffects
"sh"
"SL"

specishul

catherene
prussia
horse dont

texas

pecos
bill
cowboy
fairy tale

thed
chorus
choced
choed

•   •   •

My earliest journal entries continue to intrigue me. In the beginning, they were blunt instruments, pure and simple; my handwriting is often crammed against other people's pens, as we built off one another's attempts to communicate. It's often a dramatically condensed dialogue, where I am mainly being instructed by those around me, usually my mother or Anne. On one page, I can clearly see my own script attempting to write down the days of the week. I begin with Friday, have a major confusion at Wednesday—which I mark as "MW" and then scratch out—and I don't include a weekend at all. My mother's handwriting appears on top of mine where she inserts Saturday and Sunday in the appropriate slots.

Though some of the words I wrote down were direct responses to other people's questions, I wonder about the point at which my writing became self-generated. Even a pretty crude call and response on these pages was precious in its own right because I could rarely see or hear the words in my own head. An unwritten word was an unthought. Writing them down changed everything—alchemy itself. On a given day, I was the maker of the words *bag, cab, bear, chorus, narwhal, Nevada, Nintendo, bridge, cowboy,* and *spruce*. In the excitement of creation, it almost felt as if I summoned the words into their very being. It was as if they would never have existed in the world without my pen.

In my journals, a discovered word was a sacrament—a thing I could write. And if I could write the thing, I could read it. If I could read the thing, I could often say it. The process indicated that there was much more to explore, a rapturous language life that could be sought and, more importantly, found. When I pass over the pages now, I linger on sections containing mainly my own writing. There are exceptions, like when someone tries to phonetically correct my pronunciation, reminding me that some written words with a *c* in them can make a *sh* sound when spoken aloud, like the word *special*. But what about all of these other words? Why had my mind singled them out as important back then? I feel like an archeologist walking through ruins that are littered with the odd artifacts of an ancient city.

These are the first things I wanted to write? This is what I was thinking about when I woke up?

Words like *Sainte Chapelle* and *catacombs* appeared because I had been in Paris right before I came to Scotland. My friend Michael Krass was subletting an apartment there. But why would I write the word *jeweller* before the word *head*? Why the word *tumor* instead of the word *aneurysm*? And how could this possibly be a relevant moment to recall the Empress Catherine the Great and her rumored sexual proclivities in Prussia in the early 1700s (*cathrene prussia horse-donk*)?

I realize that the earliest words were mainly nouns—things I could visualize. Research shows that language acquisition happens similarly in a child's brain: developing minds have vocabularies that are densely populated by words for solid objects. Specifically, children seem to have a preference for things with a defined shape. Only after that, children move on to abstract concepts for intangible things, like *honor* or *trust*, and start to adopt words for their emotions. An interesting anomaly in my case is that I wrote the word *amor*, Spanish for *love*, early on. I am not sure if I even knew what the word meant as I wrote it. I had spoken nearly fluent Spanish before the rupture, but post-stroke it was worse than my English.

Regardless of why I had written these exact words down, the thing clearest to me here is that I wasn't a child, and I wasn't starting from scratch. I was a twenty-seven-year-old who had accumulated life experiences and was trying to remember, and communicate, these impressions.

I didn't use my limited writing skills to address my current emotional state, though—terms like *happy* or *sad*—or perhaps the most applicable word at the time: *confused*—never appear on these pages. That might seem especially odd to a casual observer. But when there is a neural-bleed, all the mechanisms of the organism are burdened. Every moment of existence requires new effort. Life itself is effortful. There is air to breathe, food to eat, and the basic needs of the body to fulfill. It's likely that expending energy on the emotional circuits was just a lower priority on my body's checklist. My brain had a lot to process already.

6

BJ and Laura had extended their trips to stay with me in the hospital for a while longer, but they had both reluctantly booked their tickets back to New York City by mid-September. They had obligations they could no longer ignore. BJ had his courses at Columbia University; Laura was in a new show and had already missed a few rehearsals.

A day before Laura left, she joined my mom in my hospital room, lowered the guardrail on my inclined bed, and flopped down beside me.

Lauren, I want you to know that I got in contact with Jonah, she said. I tried to reach him a lot earlier, but didn't tell you because I hadn't heard back from him. Apparently he was camping up in Alaska and didn't see any of my e-mails until now because he was completely off the grid. Which is just so . . . Jonah. Anyway, he's returned to civilization, and he really wants to be involved in what is going on here.

Jonah. How could I not have thought of him before? We had been dating for years. And Alaska. Of course. It was his summer camping trip with his old Seattle friends.

My mother crossed her arms firmly.

Jonah wants to come to the hospital, Lauren.

My mind grappled with the concept. There was a location that was not here, a time that was not now, and they could potentially collapse into each other. My parents and friends had been constants in my hospital world, like the window and the rocking chair, but they left at the end of every day. And as much as I enjoyed everyone's presence around me, I didn't exactly miss them when they were gone because I always had the companionship of the Quiet. But this was the very first time it occurred to me that someone might arrive from somewhere else. An unexpected addition.

Do you really want him here? my mother asked, her lips pursed. Of course, it's your decision to make.

I looked to her and tried to read her face like I would read Anne's during speech therapy. Was she wearing the *very good* or *not exactly* expression? Since the rupture, I had gone from naturally being able to intuit someone else's feelings to struggling to pick up on basic emotional tells. This interpersonal navigation is what psychologists call *Theory of Mind* (ToM). It is an ability that becomes manifest in most people around four or five years old, and in short, it's a person's ability to imagine what someone else might be thinking.

The easiest way to check for Theory of Mind is by conducting a *false-belief* test. To do this, you need to set up a condition that defies an expectation, like putting pencils inside a tube that usually holds candy. You ask a child: *What do you think is inside here?* The child, recognizing the tube, will usually answer: *candy*. Then, you let the pencils spill out. When you return them to the tube and ask the child again what they think is inside the tube, they will tell you: *pencils*. They've learned their lesson. But when you ask the child what someone not in the room might think is in this container, they still say pencils. It's too hard to imagine any worldview other than their own.

Many developmental psychologists say that the changes in a child's brain when they acquire Theory of Mind are directly correlated with their language skills. It's a controversial idea, but acquiring ToM skills happens around the age of major linguistic milestones, such as creating complex sentence structures to express hypothetical situations or make a counterfactual statement. It creates a thought versus reality paradigm, like *If I hadn't seen inside this tube, I would have assumed different contents, but since I have been let in on the secret* . . . and so on.

A subordinate clause can completely change the way you see the world. And in the hospital, my language skills did resemble those of a child. I lacked a lot of vocabulary, syntax, and grammar, internally and externally. I didn't possess the powers of complicated inferences. It's nearly impossible to know how much my language skills actually resembled that of a child developing language for the first time, or even if language is as imperative to ToM reasoning as some researchers suggest. But it would have explained a few things in my case. Maybe without a certain amount of language, some thoughts are unthinkable.

My mother was still looking at me, waiting for my response about Jonah.

Well, Lauren? she asked. Do you want him to come here? Yes or no?

No? I asked her.

The people in the room nodded their approval. *No* seemed to be the correct response.

The first time I ever met Jonah was at a party in a Russian restaurant on Brighton Beach, five years before the rupture. He was introduced to me as a classmate of Laura's, and we hardly spoke that night, so I didn't think much about our meeting or about him.

Until I got a phone call from him a few days later.

In the apartment I shared with Laura and BJ, we kept a communal phone in the kitchen. My roommates had recently encountered a discarded box overflowing with 1970s *Playboy* magazines on our street corner, and when we discovered a seven-page spread, a pornographic rendering of the old Mother Goose rhyme about the days of the week, we found it so delightful we festooned our breakfast nook with it. I remember being completely surrounded by these scantily clad bunnies the night Jonah called. When I heard who it was, I shouted for Laura to pick up the line.

Actually, I was calling for you, Jonah said. Confused, I briefly locked eyes with "Monday's Child"—who was full of face and then some. What was this all about?

Jonah explained that his birthday was coming up, and he wanted to know if I might be free to swing by his party. At first, I was a little perplexed by the personal invitation. I wasn't sure I could pick Jonah's face out of a crowd. But I was also intrigued, so I said I might stop by.

He called again the next day, though. He said he had decided to cancel the party.

Too much hassle, he said. But let's keep the date. We can meet at Sake Bar Decibel on St. Mark's. Do you know it?

I did. But this was a lot of newfound pressure. What kind of guy makes a first date on his birthday? I agreed to meet him, but then immediately plied Laura for more information to decide if I should back out or not. She said Jonah was the most brilliant guy in any of her classes, from scene study to physics, but "moody" didn't begin to cover his emotional swings.

Don't get me wrong; he's always been pretty nice to me, she said. But he is opinionated, often judgmental, and I'm glad I've stayed on his good side. He can be pretty intimidating.

The profile was somewhat off-putting, though I was intrigued enough not to cancel. Right before the date, I took two shots of Wild Turkey to steel me for whatever the night might have in store.

The staircase of Decibel was a repurposed fire escape, an entrance that looked more like an exit. I descended the clanging iron steps and looked around. I didn't see Jonah anywhere. So, I ordered a bottle of sake, sat in the corner, and waited.

Ten minutes passed. Then twenty. Thirty minutes in, the cute lady bartender gave me a sympathetic look and a second carafe of sake for free. By the forty-minute mark, I had nearly finished that bottle, too.

This guy had gone through all of the trouble of inviting a stranger out in this incredibly awkward way, cancelling his birthday party, only to stand her up? The possibility of not meeting him was both a relief and a disappointment. I was about to leave when a twitchy figure darted through the crowd, saw me, and froze.

What are you doing here? Jonah stammered. You weren't down here all this time, were you?

Yep, I said, bristling a little. All the time.

I was here too. He shook his head. But upstairs. I was waiting outside.

It was an especially brisk night for a New York autumn. Slightly more sympathetic to the misunderstanding, I softened my tone a little.

Well, now that we've found each other, I said, at least have some sake to warm up.

Jonah sat down and had a quick sip, but sprang back from his chair like an elastic band being snapped. He cupped his left hand over his mouth and held up his index finger, in a just-one-second gesture. Before I could completely register what was happening, he was sprinting toward the back of the restaurant. A few minutes later he came back and apologized.

I'm just nervous, he said sheepishly. Sorry I threw up.

He threw up?! Jesus. Who was this guy? Should I just leave?

But something kept me in my seat. His anxiety was oddly flattering. Jonah told me that he had admired me from afar at school. He had heard me perform some Joni Mitchell songs, had watched me in a scene from *Richard III*. He had wanted to ask me out for a long time and sounded almost starstruck.

Jonah had made a pretty eccentric entrance to this date, and I think that's why I paid close attention to everything he said and did that night. Almost immediately, I knew he was harmless. A bit of an oddball, sure, but who wasn't? He was also a bundle of incongruities. His slim and hairless build was somewhat feminine. But he was more than six feet tall, and his face was full of well-defined angles—his cheeks, chin, and jaw exhibited an unmistakable masculinity. It was easy to find him attractive. At the time, men in New York were donning the "metrosexual" look: tight jeans, plunging V-neck shirts, and oversize plastic glasses. Jonah was wearing a North Face fleece and hiking boots.

He also had an unvarnished way of describing himself. He mused about his old high school car, a conspicuously un-macho, lime-green VW Beetle with a built-in flower vase on the dashboard. He opened up about his family, too. He had a sister, a visual artist who was a little younger than him. His parents had divorced when he was a preteen, but his father had received sole custody of the kids. Jonah said this was awarded because of his mother's increasing mental instability, though the details of what actually happened seemed a bit obscure. He had been born and raised in Las Vegas, but his father moved the kids to leafy Seattle, splitting his childhood between two of the most dissimilar cities in the country. Though he and his father remained close, he'd severed ties with his mother long ago.

It was like no date I had ever been on. Jonah was showing his deck, giving me way too much information way too early. But, there was a lot I liked about him. He had uncommon stories and an uncommon way of telling them. When he started praising his cat back in Seattle, whom he had named Neutron, I teased him, asking if she had any "neutrinos."

He laughed hard at my joke. An earnest, smoker's laugh.

So much of his behavior was endearing. I'd been waiting for the difficult personality type that Laura had prepared me for, so Jonah's total lack of guile caught me off guard. I could tell immediately that he did not suffer fools lightly—he had already enumerated a few things and people he could no longer make time for, and shockingly this list had come to include his own mother. But every decision he made seemed incredibly considered, never careless, and being in the company of someone who is that discriminating has its own allure. It means that you have succeeded where so many have failed. Under Jonah's gaze that night, I started to feel resplendent.

By closing time, Jonah and I had huddled close together. I didn't open up nearly as much as he did, but his sincerity impressed me. *Intimidating* was hardly the word I would use to describe him. But as we walked out of the bar together, the flirtation from the basement was exposed to some ground-floor realities.

Jonah hesitantly asked if I was interested in going upstairs for a drink and pointed at "his place" across the street. It was a dorm. Not only was he still a student, he lived with other students. I had graduated a year earlier, and I was moving onward and upward. Or that was the plan, at least.

Though I was glad I had indulged my curiosity about Jonah, he had already proved himself both exhilarating and exhausting. So I told him thanks, but no thanks. And I said bluntly that I didn't think it could ever work out with us.

Oh. His eyes drooped. Umm. Okay.

Then, I pulled a few copies of *Playboy* I had snatched from our apartment's newest stockpile out of my bag and dropped them into Jonah's hands. His eyes were amused, but his expression completely befuddled.

For your birthday, I explained. I've got a whole box of them back at home.

He smirked. Can I at least walk you to the subway?

No need, I said, kissing his cheek. I prefer to walk alone.

Back at my apartment, I kept Jonah's phone number on my desk between my computer monitor and my trash can. I passed it often but didn't throw it out. More than a month later, Laura told me that Jonah had been moping around school since our date.

You really got under his skin, she said.

It was nice to not be so easily forgotten. More than nice. Jonah and I had established a mutual interest, and though I hadn't anticipated it would last longer than a night, it managed to linger in both of us. When I finally dialed Jonah's number, I just invited myself over to his place. There we wasted no time, giving a fervid answer to the question of what could've happened a month earlier.

Though I wasn't able to remember any of this in the hospital, this was how Jonah and I began.

A couple days after my friends left Scotland, my mother brought Jonah up again.

He keeps calling, honey. Keeps saying he wants to fly out to Scotland. And I don't know anymore. . . . Do you think it might be good to have him here?

There was a tone in her voice, a softness in her eyes. It appeared she was giving me a cue.

Yes? I asked her.

Well then, my dad said. You can speak to him yourself. He's on the phone now.

I looked up, surprised, and before I had any time to prepare myself further, my dad put his cell phone against my ear.

Lauren? Jonah's voice crackled through the line. Is that you, Lauren?

Everything about this situation was mesmerizing to me. I was holding a phone again, and even though it felt clumsy in my doll-like hand, I wasn't dropping it. And suddenly, I was walking. I was walking away from my room to the far stairway, so I could take in every transmitted syllable. Jonah was saying he missed me, he loved me, he wanted to be with me. He had probably already been briefed that the conversation would go the way it was going; that I wouldn't be an active part of our dialogue, and I wouldn't be able to reciprocate most of what he was sharing. But he talked and I listened.

Jonah sounded so sure of himself as he pitched his travel plan to me; he seemed to have considered all of the intricate aspects of his trip to Scotland in advance. I found that impressive. I was still perplexed by the simplest parts of my daily life, having difficulty imagining even five minutes into the future, and this made Jonah's certainty incredibly comforting. What do you say? Jonah asked. Do you think I can come see you? I mean, would you like that?

Yes. To everything Jonah asked, I said *Yes. Yes,* he could come. *Yes,* I would like that. It was nice to say *Yes* to Jonah, partially because we were in agreement, and partially because I was excited to say the word itself. *Yes* was one of the few parts of my vocabulary I could use with confidence.

Anticipating a future event was something I no longer had much talent for, but Jonah made me believe that his visit was something I should look forward to. And that pricked a sense of excitement in me. I walked back to my room and passed the phone back to my mom. She could manage whatever needed to be managed—travel details, calendars, addresses, telling Jonah where we would be staying, and proposing places to stay nearby. My job was done. I had said *Yes.* Everything else was up to her.

And when my mother hung up with Jonah, she reported back.

Here's the plan, kiddo. The hospital isn't going to keep you much longer, so I told Jonah to come after your release. You can spend some time together here in Scotland, and then you'll travel with me back to Los Angeles so you can recover at home.

There was a lot of information packed in her statement, and it was unclear to me how I should receive it. I absorbed it all piece by piece, like the knock of the rocking chair hitting the plaster wall.

Release. Boom.

Recover. Boom.

Home. Boom.

7

Ever since Alison and Alan Paterson had welcomed my parents into their home, my folks had taken to calling them "The Angels of Edinburgh." The Patersons had a well lived-in house, which made it easy to relax. The drawers in the kitchen stuck. Plates were left in the sink and board games were scattered around communal spaces. It was the house of a university professor and a schoolteacher, so in nearly every room books and papers were piled on chairs and desks, and even fought for dominance on stretches of the floor. Two of the three children had already left the nest, and lucky for all of us, their empty rooms had accommodated the influx of unexpected houseguests that summer. The Patersons remained good-humored and unreasonably kind during our long occupation. I was in the hospital most of that time, but my mother told me about how one day, she had accidentally dropped a hot iron on the Patersons' wall-to-wall carpeting, and while my mom had been mortified, Alison had simply laughed it off. She assured my mother there was some spare carpet in a closet somewhere.

All of us came to enjoy the company of the youngest son in the family, the one who was still living at home. He was a cheery eighteen-year-old who shared my brother's name: Michael. BJ, Laura, and I had met him our first night in Edinburgh—and it had been a memorable meeting because it started with a pretty major case of mistaken identity. Alan had picked us up from the train station, and when we arrived at the house, we were invited to the kitchen for a homemade dinner. This was when I saw another figure in the room. He was hunched over a stool, shoving the remains of a digestive biscuit into his mouth.

It was my brother.

Beyond shocked, I blurted out, How on earth did *you* get here?!

When the boy looked directly at me, it was clear it wasn't my brother at all. It was the red hair, the transparent, freckled skin, and the posture that threw me. As he stood up straight to dust off the crumbs from his trousers, I realized Michael Paterson was slimmer and taller than my brother. BJ and Laura remarked on the resemblance, too, but I found the physical similarities so striking that I never really took to calling him Michael, instead using his nickname, "Materson." You can't call twins the same name, after all. Our group spent a lot of time with Materson, especially after he had insisted on making us an English specialty: banoffee pie. The gesture was so kind, from a teenage boy no less, that our affection for him increased exponentially.

My parents were equally delighted to meet my brother's doppelgänger when they arrived in Scotland and soon adopted his nickname, too. I assume his general presence made them feel comfortable, more like they were at home.

It was late September when I was released from the hospital, and as I was moving back into the Paterson house, my father was leaving it. He needed to go back to LA. My parents' advertising agency was small—my father was the only writer on staff, and my mother was the CEO—and their clients were getting restless. It was harder to see my dad leave than Laura or BJ, but it was clear that he was more upset about the departure than I was. He apologized to me profusely, explaining and re-explaining the situation, until my mother assured him that she and I were going to be just fine, and he could always trust the women in our household to take care of themselves.

It was a weekday morning in the Paterson kitchen, and Mom and I were alone in the house. I sat with a cup of tea at the table, while Mom washed dishes at the sink.

Then, there was a knock—the sound I had forgotten to be expecting.

When I opened the front door, the sky was grey and everything around me was a little out of focus. The pale man on the step was almost fully obscured by the overgrown lavender bush situated just below the Patersons' front step. He was dressed all in brown, a brown vest with matching brown pants and jacket, but his grey-blue eyes were sharp. We were frozen there in a stretched and shapeless pause. And then, in slow motion, he started to extend his arms toward me. The tweed of his jacket scratched my exposed neck, snapping me back to attention.

Jonah. This was Jonah. I had seen him only a month ago in New York, but that month might as well have been a lifetime.

Look at you, up and walking around! I didn't think they'd keep your hair! He smiled and let his eyes tour my body. Good God, Lauren, I'm so glad to see you. Missed you so much. Jonah gave me a hug and then lightly stroked my cheek.

The hairs on my arms jolted up when Jonah initiated this more intimate contact. My alarmed skin bristled in goose bumps. I took a moment or two to relax into the touch, and then I even started to enjoy it. But Jonah was touching me like we were having a long-delayed reunion, and the sensations he brought out in me felt much more like a blind date. Outside of this interaction, the flow of my mind was still mainly Quiet, and though Jonah's arrival pleased me, the introduction of this person into my new world was something I approached tentatively. Would it change the peace I'd been experiencing? I knew what Jonah had been in the past: the boyfriend. But for the time being he was just a familiar stranger.

Jonah took my hand, and continued to hold it as we went into the house. As he and my mother spoke in the kitchen, I struggled to remember if they had met before. I was getting better at reading faces—sad versus happy, fatigued versus energized—but that was the extent of my emotional intelligence. My mother's expression during the conversation was much harder for me to tease apart. She had been introduced to Jonah a few times over the years, never forming a strong opinion, but when I was actually in crisis, she had zero patience for someone who didn't leap into action on my behalf. Being off the grid on a camping trip hadn't exempted Jonah from that expectation. I don't know how much of her intense protectiveness Jonah could sense, or if he felt judged by her, because below their pleasantries, the two were probably sizing each other up. But I was oblivious to it at the time. The only thing I remember feeling about this conversation was that people talked a little too much.

Jonah told my mother of his love of traveling. He reminded her that he and I had been to Europe before, on a vacation to Switzerland and Italy two and a half years ago. Maybe this was his sly way of giving his credentials and competence, hinting that he and I might be able to venture off safely together, without a chaperone. My mother was initially hesitant, but eventually admitted that walking around on our own couldn't be too dangerous.

As I started to pick up my wire-bound journal from the table, Mom explained its significance to Jonah.

When Lauren has trouble saying words, she'll try to write them down. It usually helps.

Jonah and I went into the city later that day, but I hadn't expected that the cobblestones and inclines would exhaust me the way they did. The Fringe Festival was now over and the town was much sleepier. With Laura and BJ, I had always been on the move. Now, I had to rest every block, a sitting tour of Edinburgh. But Jonah never complained. When he wasn't acting in New York, he worked as a children's tutor and taught English as a second language, a skill set that was quickly put to use with me. As we walked around town, we played a prolonged word game he had employed before. It was a bit more active than Laura's prompt sheet, and it was as simple as it was effective, especially since I was able to use the journal the whole time. I wrote down words that all began with the same letter. My journal pages mention *New Zealand* to *Neanderthal*, and later, *Hammurabi*, *Huntington*, and *Humphrey Bogart*. Jonah's encouragement made me laugh.

I loved how imaginative the game was, and I especially appreciated that he never asked me to recall personal details of my former life, something I was still having a lot of difficulty with. I felt Jonah, more than anyone else, was willing to interact in the present tense with me. We were in this new world, moment to moment, and we were there together.

Back at the Patersons' home, we collapsed in their living room, me in the armchair and him on the couch until he scooped me up in his arms and placed me on his lap.

You're going to have to indulge this irresistible urge I have to kiss you, he said, before laying dozens of pecks on the backs of my arms and shoulders.

Watch out, Lauren, I might never stop.

What was Jonah expecting from me next? I pivoted my upper body to face him, and unclear what he might want, I experimented by kissing him squarely on the mouth. The short exchange was gummy and taut. Since I had kept my lips closed, it tasted like nothing, like air inside of a balloon. I pulled back to gauge his response.

Is this okay? I asked.

Of course, Lauren. Of course this is okay. This is good.

And I agreed that it was good, but it was also very, very peculiar. Jonah circled his arms around my waist, resting his cheek against my back. He hugged me and I hugged the journal.

8

After two weeks back at the Patersons' home, it was approaching October, and we were readying to return to the US. The neurosurgeons had instructed my mother not to let me travel from Edinburgh to Los Angeles on a single flight because they wanted me to spend as little time as possible in the restrictive air pressure of a plane cabin. Taking their advice, my mother booked tickets to California with a three-day layover in New York.

Before we left, Jonah and I shared a bench in the Patersons' backyard. My face was following the sun, and my neck was resting on Jonah's collarbone. There was a strong sense of order inside me. I felt the intricate and ineffable everywhere. The same patterns that contained the bird on the ledge and the worm guzzling the soil were the same patterns that contained the weight of my head and the shape of Jonah's shoulder. I couldn't describe this sense of symmetry, but all was as it should be.

After a while, I broke my silence, mentioning something to Jonah that probably took him by surprise.

I am not afraid to die, I said.

My sentence structure was still very shaky. I doubt I was able to qualify or contextualize the comment much. But I didn't feel I had to because I had never said anything that true.

It's all going to be okay. You are not about to die, Lauren, Jonah said, while tightening his grip on me. You don't need to worry about it anymore.

But I'm not worried at all, I said. That's what I'm trying to tell you.

I wasn't sure Jonah heard me, or if he understood that I didn't need any comfort then. Quite the opposite. But his body relaxed a bit and he said: Wish we could stay in this garden forever. You, me, and the bumblebees. He sighed. Don't get me wrong—I'm glad we'll get to spend some time in New York together too. It's just more peaceful here, more authentic somehow. But, then again, everything feels more real when you leave New York City.

Returning to New York didn't much matter to me, but my mother thought it would be nice to pick up some things from my apartment, and maybe see some friends while I was in town.

Could be fun, she said. We can throw a brunch or something; make the whole day an open house. People can wander in and out to wish you well. I agreed to the plan and Jonah helped me write the e-mail.

My own apartment was being sublet, but my friend Rachel had offered up her place for us to use. She and her husband were out of town, but they had left a key and told us to use the house as if it were our own. When we arrived stateside, Jonah returned to his apartment in Brooklyn, and Mom and I headed to Rachel's apartment on the Upper East Side, where we both fell into a deep—and much needed—sleep.

The next day I got up early, initially disoriented by waking up in Rachel's bedroom. It was the morning of the party and still dark outside. My mom was asleep on the other side of the wide bed, and the sky over the East River was showing the pink thumbprints of dawn. It felt like a lucky day already.

Laura and BJ arrived with orange juice, baguettes, and a bouquet of flowers, and quickly got to work assisting my mom, who had decided to assemble a large egg scramble. Jonah appeared soon after that, looking a little groggy. I hadn't thought about the details of the party beforehand, but once friends started arriving, I was overjoyed. These people. I had forgotten I knew these people. And even though I couldn't remember many details of who they were or how we knew each other, the recognition was instinctual and reassuring. There was my best friend from high school, Grace, who had moved from California to New York to do her graduate work at Columbia. There was Michael Krass, the friend and former NYU professor with whom I stayed in Paris right before the Edinburgh Fringe Festival. In a bright yellow dress I borrowed from Rachel's closet, I sat on the far corner of the couch, the end point of a receiving line of former classmates and castmates. Every kind word or touch sent me into tiny spasms of grace. There couldn't have been more than ten people in the room at any given time, but the voices soared and tumbled around me in a blissful din. People looked luminous to me, better and brighter than themselves, more like constellations. I started to feel as if I were rising from the couch, hovering closer and closer to the ceiling fixtures, and when a friend lightly clasped onto my arm, I was thankful for his anchor because it felt that I might otherwise have drifted away in unspeakable delight.

However, as more people continued to arrive in waves, the aural bombardment became too intense. I went to Rachel's bedroom to lie down. I still wanted everyone to stay, to eat, to talk, but I couldn't appreciate the celebration unless I was behind the closed door. I splayed out like a pressed daffodil between the white sheets of Rachel's bed, trying to stop my heart from racing. I didn't mind if people entered the bedroom, as long as they knocked on the door, came in one at a time, and spoke quietly. For the next two hours, I'd doze in between visits. The bright, lucky party was happening just outside this room and that was just as I wanted it.

But then I threw up. And I kept throwing up.

When my mother came to check on me, her expression quickly morphed into what I had come to identify as "worry." I didn't think my sickness was a major cause for concern or worth stopping the party for. I argued that I was fine, but my point was somewhat weakened when I leaned over to vomit again into an empty Duane Reade bag.

My mom called my old doctor's office back in LA. She tried to remain calm, but when the nurse on call told her that vomiting could be an early sign of neurological crisis, she went into disaster management mode.

I tried one more time to find enough language to protest, to assure her that I really wasn't feeling that bad, but my mom insisted we go to the ER immediately. She helped me out of Rachel's dress and into some yoga pants. We hopped into a cab and several people from the party followed close behind.

When we arrived at the nearest hospital, my mother explained my recent medical situation and I was treated before anyone else there—express IV, express consult. After the exam, though, the doctors decided that I had most likely caught a strain of flu on the plane back from Edinburgh, nothing more. It was a common problem for people who had stayed in sterile environments for long stretches. The doctors asked me to stay for observation overnight, just in case, but my friends were still milling about the hospital waiting room with bagels and opened bottles of champagne. As soon as it was clear that I was in no imminent danger, they renewed their celebration with vigor. And my mom got herself settled into a hotel room next door.

Unfortunately for everyone who saw me that morning, enthusiasm wasn't the only thing that was contagious. My bug proved especially virulent, and most of them quickly fell ill, no one as badly as my poor mother. When I was released from the hospital, she had planned to join Jonah and me on a trip to my Brooklyn apartment, but her illness kept her from going anywhere. Instead, she gave me explicit instructions: gather any clothes and items I might need in LA and hurry back.

My apartment in Greenpoint was a two bedroom that I was sharing with a journalism grad student from Australia. Built in the 1940s, the ceilings of the charming third-floor apartment were high, the walls were thick, and none of the windows faced the busy street. The living room looked out over an unused garden. It was the most relaxing home I'd ever lived in.

But for reasons I couldn't exactly pinpoint then, this feeling of calm didn't wash over me as Jonah and I opened the front door. All I saw was the pile of unwashed dishes in the sink and two lightbulbs out in the hallway. I felt sick all over again.

Maybe those stairs were a little too much exertion, Jonah said, concerned. Do you want to lie down for a while? No one is going to mind.

It sounded like a good idea initially, but I quickly fixated on the fact that a stranger's sheets were on my bed. Everything smelled off. I didn't feel I belonged there at all. I rushed to stuff a suitcase and did so with very little care about what I packed. I was going to California to recover. How many pairs of underwear would I need for that?

Getting to Los Angeles proved more complicated than initially planned. The bouts of sickness my mother and I battled through delayed our return, so we were still staying in the hotel near the hospital when Rachel returned to New York. She hurried over to visit us, catching a yellow cab straight from JFK.

Jonah and I were in the deli below the hotel, picking up more ginger ale for my mother. I caught sight of Rachel getting out of a taxi, wrestling with her unwieldy suitcase. As soon as she spotted me, she dropped all of her bags in a heap and pulled me into a tight, perfumed hug.

There you are! she said. There's the Lauren I know and love.

Rachel didn't mean to upset me, but I found her statement profoundly jarring. I didn't jerk away from her embrace, but inwardly I was recoiling. I had woken up from brain surgery changed—there was me, here and now, but I sensed there was another shadowy character in the mix here too: The Girl I Used to Be. I couldn't easily access the memories of this girl in any complete way and wasn't actively engaging in her senses of attachment or desire. I didn't know if I wanted what she used to want, or if I cared about what she used to care about. And, strangely enough, I wasn't mourning the loss of that past self. She was simply gone, which was neither a good nor a bad thing. The life I was living suited me fine. But somehow Rachel hadn't seen the chasm between those two people at all, and it was the misidentification that wounded me. Under this unforgiving spotlight, it became clear that this issue of "not belonging" wasn't limited to my experience being inside my old apartment, it was also permeating my interactions with my family and friends. The Girl I Used to Be was someone I didn't know, but with whom everyone else was on intimate terms. I felt a kind of warmth between Rachel and me, an unidentifiable affection that must have been forged in years of friendship, but I certainly was not the Lauren who Rachel knew and loved. And I might never be that person again. Wasn't that transformation obvious? Didn't it radiate off my very skin? In that moment, though, I wasn't able to explain to Rachel how I was feeling. I didn't even try. Only later, I confided my concerns to my journal.

> *Rachel. "There's soul." "Youre*
> *right here" Why?*
> *Thats is no there?*

I tried to transcribe my interaction with Rachel, word-for-word, into my journal. I had graduated from scratching isolated words onto a page to some fragile sentence constructions. I wasn't able to know how fractured these sentences really were, but somehow I did sense I wasn't able to put down Rachel's words exactly.

I had acquired this other woman's family and friends, her boyfriend and apartment. What to make of this familiar unfamiliarity? I was not the girl who had built this life and shaped it to her personal preferences. Though I didn't have any major complaints about what I had encountered yet, I also didn't know how to interact with it, or what my obligations might be to the system I had been inserted into. Did I just accept this inheritance, with all its fearful and joyful dimensions? Did I have any say in the matter? Would I ever feel anything like The Girl I Used to Be? And was that something I should even want?

I didn't know how to know. I didn't know how to remember.

SEPTEMBER

PART TWO

HOMECOMING

*I have a feeling I'm falling / on rare occasions / but most of the time I
have my feet on the ground / I can't help it if the ground itself is falling.*
LAWRENCE FERLINGHETTI

1

The disorientation might have begun on the freeways that crisscrossed Los Angeles or on the streets that led up into the hills of Altadena. Maybe it began in the driveway of my parents' California Spanish home, lit from within. Whenever it began, the feeling could no longer be ignored as I walked out of the mild September night and into my family's kitchen. The smell of roasted chicken in the stove curdled against the tang of bleach coming from the laundry room. A host of chrome appliances ticked and chirped as electricity buzzed through them. The pale wood floorboards and the still life on the wall suddenly seemed like co-conspirators against my sense of balance. The entire house was humming.

My dad and grandma were there, waiting for me with open arms, but I couldn't fully match their embraces. I needed a place to situate myself again, to reconnect with the Quiet. The bathtub upstairs seemed ideal. But as I lowered my body into the steaming water, vague memories of every bath I had ever taken in that room started to populate the tub. There was the time with the inflatable white pillow, and another time, long after the pillow had popped. There were baths when I'd kept my feet planted on the floor of the tub, and others when I'd let my legs float. Some when I submerged my head with my hair swaying like seaweed, and others when I hadn't wet my hair at all. This was not the relaxing dip I had hoped it would be. The bath was too damn crowded.

I focused on the garbage can, which began to shape-shift before my eyes. What was it doing? Where was it going? Its unanticipated animation was unsettling, but there was a terrible beauty in the hallucination, too. The only thing I came to fear more than the kaleidoscopic display was the possibility that the splendor might one day stop.

Over the next few weeks, in search of silence and to subdue the clamor, I preferred to be alone in the house. I kept the TVs and radios off. I didn't pick up a ringing phone unless I had to. I sat in undecorated hallways or lay in the backyard, beneath the sprawling net of tree limbs. With my ears in the rough grass, I'd single out the blades that had been spared by the gardener. Then, the Quiet would find me.

And in my journal, I wondered: Would this house ever stop becoming?

> *every rgorm. different.*
> *make kaleidscope. new sparts*
> *every time. will this house*
> *keep on becom̶eimg. How many*
> *rime can i surprised by the*
> *trasht can*

From the kitchen table, I could see my grandmother tottering down the driveway from the little house in the backyard. She had a round, heavyset build; her gait betrayed her arthritis and the subtle pain in every step. But while her body had lost its fortitude, her mind was as keen as ever. She had been a nurse for fifty years, and now into her early eighties, she remained an avid reader, easily finishing a book a day. She would enlist family members to make weekly trips to the local library to keep up with her demand. To join me in the main house, my grandmother needed only to go up the single stair that entered into the kitchen. But it was not so simple for her. She would have to grip the doorjamb with one hand and use her free hand to balance her book, her cup of coffee, and whatever else she was carrying around. She moved like a seesaw and entered most rooms sideways. I didn't get up from my seat while she enacted this elaborate procedure in front of me because, even when it was a very unsteady day, she didn't like people to help her.

Not long after she retired from being a nurse in rural Montana, my grandmother moved in with my parents in Los Angeles. That little cottage in the backyard, sometimes referred to as the "granny shack," had been built specifically for her relocation. Though she was my maternal grandmother, my father never treated her like an in-law. As soon as he would wake up every day, he'd freshly grind dark roasted beans, and would usually hand-deliver her morning cup of black coffee.

Hey punkin, she greeted me warmly, lurching toward the sink, where she deposited her coffee cup.

As my grandmother joined me at the kitchen table, she surveyed the contents of the care packages that had amassed there: a stuffed elephant, a box of markers, a plastic jack-o-lantern full of microwave popcorn, and romantic comedies starring Sarah Jessica Parker. And there were so many letters, many from people I hardly knew, but all addressed to me. Gram patted my arm, her touch soft as a peach.

It's like Queen for a Day in here, she said. How does it feel to get so much attention, honey?

Feel? I didn't feel anything about it. Was I supposed to? I'd left most of the gifts unopened and the cards unread. They all said the same thing anyway: *Get well soon.* The whole concept was baffling to me.

In general, I was a bit unsure if I was using the right words, in the right order, whenever I was speaking. But it was different whenever I interacted with my grandmother. She always managed to understand me. Why do you think people keep sending me these things, Gram?

It's because you are a miracle, she said.

But I haven't done anything, I protested.

Well, she said, and thought about my statement for a little longer. For being a survivor then, she concluded finally.

I looked toward the cards again. *Get Well.* The phrasing sounded odd to me. Like: Get a Seat or Get a Spoon. Was *well* something you could *get*? And didn't these people know that I was out of the hospital and that everything was clearly fine?

But I am well already, I told her.

She considered my comment carefully. You know, punkin, you don't seem too upset about being uprooted from your boyfriend and school, and your whole life on the other side of the country. And that's good. I'm so pleased you're not letting this whole situation get you down—proud that you've got the grit and constitution for this kind of thing. Still, I've got something gnawing on me, she said. She fixed her gaze squarely on me and I could see my reflection framed perfectly in her owl-like glasses.

The only thing that really concerns *me* about your case is that it doesn't seem to concern *you.*

2

The last moment I had shared with Jonah in New York was just outside my mother's hotel room. We had gone to the elevator together, and as we waited there, he leaned over and kissed me. I tried to follow his lead. Considering our pre-rupture timeline, Jonah and I had shared thousands of kisses through the years. Some tender, some joyful, some illicit. But I didn't feel the weight of our history then. Also, I was about to leave the state for an indefinite amount of time; I could easily have worried about our future or felt concerned that this might be our final kiss. But this also wasn't the case. It was astonishing how unpracticed I felt while kissing Jonah, and mainly I just kept hoping I was doing it right.

And the next day, I was three thousand miles away.

On a morning in late September, my mother was darting around the kitchen, trying to rush out to work. She snatched a file of papers from the counter, but an idea bubbled up in her mind that quickly registered on her face. She dashed to consult the family calendar hanging on the pantry door.

Jonah's birthday is coming up soon, isn't it? she asked me. Uh-huh. October first, it seems. Are you planning on sending him anything? A gift of some kind?

Sure, I said. It sounded like a good idea. I must have been the person who had added the date on the calendar in the first place, but there also was no way I could have remembered the event without my mother's reminder. So, what does Jonah like? I asked her.

How would I know what Jonah likes? My mother scoffed. I'm not the one who's been dating him for the last five years.

Something in my expression must have looked pitiful or confused because it stopped my mother dead in her tracks. She slowed down and sat next to me.

Oh honey, I didn't mean to be harsh, she said. It's just that you and Jonah always kept your relationship pretty private. Which was fine, and I respected your independence, but that bond didn't really include your family and friends. I was glad I could spend some time with him in Scotland, but it just wasn't enough time to know the things he really likes.

Since I wasn't allowed to drive anywhere at this stage of my recovery, my mother suggested we make Jonah some birthday cookies together when she returned that evening. In the meantime, I could try to put together some kind of care package for him. Lately, I had some experience receiving these presents in the mail, so I set about trying to prepare one myself.

My mom kept a stash of knickknacks in the house, small generic gifts in case of an unexpected occasion or unannounced visitor. For Jonah, I selected a carton of Chinese fortune sticks, still wrapped in cellophane. But I wanted to put something more precious in there too. If I packed up something that I wanted back at some point, it was like making a promise for a future meeting. I chose a music box that had been my favorite as a child. It was a wooden figurine, carved in the shape of a girl, with painted-on hair, standing on a plastic pedestal. She would be my emissary.

There was a small amount of space left in the care package. I thought of something that would fit perfectly there. On a recent walk through my neighborhood, I had seen an exquisite desert bush in full flower. Its beauty was stupefying. The plant was covered in vibrant red-orange bulbs, each the size of an avocado, the color and shape of a human heart. I left the house and walked back to where I'd seen it. It didn't bother me much that it was in a neighbor's yard. With so much surplus on this plant, a single bloom couldn't possibly be missed.

But when I grabbed for the fruit, the gesture came with a naked thump of pain. White needles spread across my palm like fur. I hadn't remembered the word *cactus* until one pricked me. As I plucked every stinging whisker, the word throbbed its way back into my vocabulary, scorching as a sunburn. By the time I drafted Jonah's birthday card, I had a greater sense of practicality. I shouldn't send this cactus bulb anywhere. It was too beautiful to dispose of, though, so I kept it for myself, handling it with gloves. I would still share it with Jonah, but a picture of it would have to suffice.

w/ Jonah
- "August 24, call my new birthday"
"You can just change your birthday. Your birthday is your birthday"
"Hey, new ~~life~~ new brain, new life, I might think on it."
Daydreaming by new birthday
Was my labor difficult? How long? How many doctors
nearby, Who ~~were~~ the ones who ne waked ~~waked wak~~ up in t the
(artful?) ~~nightmare~~ to delivery to the helpless merringone
al whole ~~year~~ minute ~~little~~ (small) ~~Lauren~~ me (insensible)

A few days later, Jonah called me while he was opening his birthday present. He ate a macaroon into the receiver.

They are still soft, he said, licking his fingers. It's adorable the way you packaged each cookie in its own Saran Wrap pocket.

I didn't need to do that? I asked.

Lauren, no one *needs* to do that, he said. But it's sweet as hell. How am I going to top this for your birthday?

I don't know, I said, giggling. Now that I have two of them.

I heard his lighter flip open.

Come again? he asked, after his first drag.

Well, waking up from a brain surgery is like a birth, I said. New brain, new life.

Sort of . . . Jonah sounded unconvinced.

I had been only slightly serious when I made the comment, but after Jonah disputed it, I realized that I really believed it. The birth and neurointervention took place in the same location (a hospital), had the same cast of characters (doctors and patients), and pretty much the same conflict (expectant parents and their mewling, helpless delivery). The Girl I Used to Be was born on a summer day, twenty-seven years ago, and I felt no attachment whatsoever to that occasion, that other life. So I tried to explain to Jonah that August 24 was much more my birthday than June 19.

I get the symbolic value. Jonah exhaled his smoke slowly into the receiver. Because the surgery was a big deal, but your birthday is your birthday, Lauren. You don't get to change that.

His dismissal was so off-putting that I stopped trying to discuss the subject. I had forgotten this aspect of Jonah's personality. He always spoke his mind, and though he could eventually change his opinion on an issue at some point, he refused to do so in the course of a conversation. The Girl I Used to Be might have been a lot like that, too. In the years before the rupture, Jonah and I had established a dynamic that was often fast-paced and competitive. When we would see an exhibit at the MoMA or watch a play at New York Theatre Workshop, we would often disagree with each other afterward. Seeing the work was the first act, discussing it was the second. We would state our claims and our interaction for hours would be all about who made the most salient point of the night. Though this pattern may not have been conducive to a supportive relationship, there were many moments of love and tenderness between us. But in a peculiar way, we tended to be at our most generous when we were not right in front of each other.

Alone in his apartment in Brooklyn Heights, or in his dad's place in Seattle, Jonah took it upon himself to narrate and record full books-on-tape for me. Knowing I liked a good story, he recorded *The Catcher in the Rye*, *Free Fall*, and *Lying Awake* in their entirety. These projects took dozens of hours to complete, and he had no editing materials or digital software. It was an old-fashioned tape recorder and this do-it-yourself quality added to the projects' charm. Sometimes a car alarm would go off, or a cat would wander into the room and meow. And I liked how all of those interruptions became a part of the permanent record, too. As much as I enjoyed the stories themselves, it was in these unrehearsed moments that I was reminded why Jonah and I had come together and stayed together. He was at his most unguarded when he recorded them, and when I listened to them, my defenses were lowered as well. He was just a man in a room making a gift for the woman he loved. I found nothing quite so beautiful as the sound of him turning the page. I tried to make him a few recordings myself, reading short excerpts from Calvino's *Invisible Cities* or Kipling's *Just So Stories*, but I didn't have the stamina for his marathon sessions. There was a lot of mutual admiration infused into these affectionate exchanges. Still, our passion never ran hotter than when we were deep in debate.

But now, only a little more than a month after the aneurysm's rupture, I wasn't able to engage with Jonah in the way I used to. I couldn't be as combative or eloquent. I didn't feel I could defend my positions in real time. When I mentioned having a second birthday, I needed eye contact, gestures, and touch to feel I was being understood. With none of that at my disposal, I simply abandoned the point.

3

My language skills were fractured and I had a radically short attention span for most topics, so there were many things I was simply unable to think about, let alone manage. Chief among those was my own medical care.

Two different ambulances had sped me to two different hospitals in Edinburgh the night of my aneurysm. There was the CT scan, the brain operation, the Doppler ultrasounds to my head. There had been medications: the morphine in the intensive unit, the nimodipine to prevent vasospasms, Albutamol and Seretide for my preexisting asthma, the tramadol, paracetamol, and dihydrocodeine to combat any breakthrough pain. There was round-the-clock monitoring, with meals doled out several times a day. If I had been a Scottish citizen, all of this care would have been free of charge. But I wasn't. Though my parents made their gratitude clear and maintained that no price tag could be too high to save their daughter's life, they still had quietly worried about how they would pay for all of it. If this treatment had been in the United States, they calculated it could easily cross over the million-dollar mark. Would they have to sell the house?

When the bill finally arrived from Scotland, they were stunned. We were expected to pay four thousand US dollars, and could do so with a payment plan as long as we needed it to be. My mother's relief commingled with her incredulity.

Four thousand dollars is no chump change, she said to my dad. But if this had been in the US? Not a chance. Four thousand dollars would've just been payment one.

But paying off old bills wasn't the only medical issue we were faced with. Dr. Salman had informed my parents that the first three months after the onset of aphasia were the most crucial for language rehabilitation, and that I would need structured therapy during this period to ensure a successful recovery going forward. But we were sliding between two medical systems on two different continents, and finding the right care was hardly streamlined. In mid-October my mother set up an appointment with a neurologist, a woman who had once helped her with her migraines.

Dr. Reiko Russin was a short woman with a greying black bob and a clipped manner of speaking. After a quick physical check, similar to the ones given to me in Scotland, my mother and I headed into her dim office.

Lauren's motor neurological exam is unremarkable, Dr. Russin said, looking severe behind her glossy oak desk.

And that's bad? My mother sounded concerned.

No, Dr. Russin replied, taking out her prescription pad. Unremarkable is good. Unremarkable is what we want. Suzanne, I'm giving you the name of some speech and language programs to consider here in the LA area. But you have to realize that Lauren is at a critical juncture at this moment, and the recovery of her full language is not yet certain. I was in the backseat of this conversation, noticing the way the doctor talked past me as if I were not in the room. Although the information she was giving seemed somewhat dire, her professional tone was reassuring.

You need to start your search for a speech therapist, Dr. Russin said, ripping the paper off the pad and handing it to my mother. She shot a steely glance in my direction and concluded: pronto.

Later that night, Jonah suggested that I might not just need a language therapist, but a regular therapist as well. He reminded me that before my injury, I had told him time and again I'd never be part of the "boomerang generation," adult children returning to their parents' home. Now that you have to be there, he said, you are bound to be feeling some psychological strain at the moment.

I reflected on his statement. Not really, I said. I don't think so, anyway.

To be on the safe side, Jonah gave me the details of a psychologist he knew out in LA, who specialized in dreams. I had never been to a therapist before and I didn't start then, either, but Jonah's mention of dreams drew my attention because they had started to feel especially important in my language recovery.

I haven't encountered extensive research about the role sleep can play in cases of aphasia per se, but there is a wealth of studies indicating that sleep assists in urgent problem solving and memory consolidation. In Scotland, I could easily sleep for eighteen hours a day, but that rest was fitful and dreamless. That changed back in California. There, going to sleep became productive. The moments right after I woke every morning were a broken hydrant of language. The people, the places, the fantastic situations all created a dynamism of recollection for me, and when I opened my eyes, I'd find a torrent of words spilling out of my pen, things I hadn't been able to remember before going to bed.

Writing down my dreams was easily the most productive time of every day.

Dream

Dreams has been to much. jumble. Interesting. Stout now. After one month.

Momument. Like Rushmore. Bigger. Older. Treacherous. With less tools on dangerous angles. Made by the Chouktow Indians. I was on the face truly true face. on the massive feet. I look on to the view. Terrifying but breath exhilating.

I feet I was afraid. a lot of precipes. Political (ally (?)) rally (?) I was talk to new people. One was famous astor. actor. I actors are phonieys. Heard the speaker. Did not see it. A precipes. ~~New~~ *Near cliffs, no guard rail And elevators. I walled With dad? (Smtimes) Get closer down, but still . . . he would preten to fall but I moved mhimia. I though he will fall a in the middle after pretending.*

The writing in the early journals, whether detailing dreams or not, gives me valuable insight into the predictable language mistakes I was un-wittingly making daily, even though I couldn't recognize them in real time. In the dream of Mount Rushmore, I had written *stout* (instead of *start*), *rally* (instead of *ally*), *wall* (instead of *walk*)—these are all *phonemic* errors, a common occurrence with people who have sustained damage to their Broca's area. These are words that sound similar, usually with the same number of syllables and vowel arrangements, but mean very different things.

Like *before* and *perform*.

Despite the fact that my parents didn't act onstage anymore, performance was part of the very fabric of my family. In the Rushmore dream, my father was playing a clown. But he was clumsy. In the dream, I kept trying to remind him that a fake punch could accidentally land as a real punch, and a stage tumble could become a critical injury, especially with the sheer precipices around him. Like it had been for me on the platform at Priscilla's Bar, it was too easy to have an actual fall in the middle of all that pretending.

4

The doorbell rang a little before noon. When I answered, there was a woman with a jet-black bouffant, thick eyeliner, and a dark lip stain standing on the threshold.

Well hello, little lady. Sorry to intrude like this but I'm an old friend of your momma's, she said in a thick Southern drawl. Knew you when you were yay-high.

The woman's lips smiled mauve as she handed me a purple orchid.

I'm just so pleased you're doing so good, honey. We've been praying hard. I can't stay, unfortunately, but you just be sure to tell your daddy how much we all appreciated his e-mails.

I thanked her for the flower, though I thought her comment was strange. Thinking it might just be post-rupture confusion, I asked my mom about it when she got home.

Well, your dad started writing these sort of . . . letters . . . as soon as we arrived in Scotland, she said. When you were still in the intensive care unit.

Oh, I said. He was writing about me, then?

Think about it, Lauren. How else could your friends have known what was going on? Not like you were able to update them yourself.

I realized my mother was right. I hardly had an online life at all; I wasn't using any social media, and would go weeks before opening an e-mail. I didn't feel like I was missing out on anything, though. I wasn't especially interested in what was going on with other people because I was too overwhelmed with what was going on with myself. And, logistically, it took too long to read an e-mail or online post. And if I wanted to answer them, I usually would need some help in doing so. I just didn't see that appeal.

But what about my friends? I asked. How did you get ahold of them?

Oh that, she said. Laura guessed your e-mail password. We've been managing all of your communications coming in and out since.

She explained that since Grace was also a PhD student in New York, they had been forwarding all my grad school business to her. While she had been managing all my official correspondence, my parents had been handling my personal letters.

I thought your father would have stopped writing these group e-mails by this point, but . . .

Wait, I said. Dad is still sending out the e-mails? These updates . . . on *me*?

Well, yeah, my mom answered, a little cautiously. But not that often anymore. Your dad just tends to overshare in the digital realm, you know?

And at that point, she admitted to me that my father's notes were not just going to my closest friends and other students in my PhD program, but also to our neighbors, ex-neighbors, family members, employees, former employees, and some of their business associates.

I was aghast, and it must have showed.

I'll make sure he stops, honey, my mother promised. Privacy has always mattered a little more to you than to your dad.

An intense reliance on others had begun the second I collapsed in Priscilla's Bar. Nurses washed me and changed my catheter, and my parents hovered over me every second I was in sight. They had brought me home and provided me with whatever I needed. Still, remarkably, the concept of *privacy* didn't occur to me until my mother uttered the word, and *speaking for* me felt very different than *doing things for* me. I needed to know what my father had been writing. What had been said on my behalf?

My father's laptop was on the dining room table, and I discovered that he had left his e-mail inbox open. When I typed the word *Scotland* into the search field, dozens of messages popped up. I chose one at random, dated September 6:

> "She can't wait to get out. Out. Out! OUT! 'I want to not be here,'
> she pouts, spreading her arms wide, eyes rolling. Syntax may be a
> little shaky, but the meaning is crystal clear. 'Here' is exactly where
> she wants to not be, thank you very much. She's fed up with hospital
> life. She's fed up with what she's being fed."

How long did it take me to read that first letter? I have no idea if it was twenty minutes or two hours, but I do know that my father's descriptions didn't align with my memories at all. Fed up with the food? I remember eating whatever was put in front of me. Fed up with hospital life? This had been fewer than two months earlier, and I knew how difficult it had been for me to even imagine any place besides the hospital. My dad said my meanings had been crystal clear to others, but how could that possibly be if he himself misunderstood me?

I was even more surprised at his characterization of my expressive aphasic symptoms:

> "Her mispronunciations and torturing of innocent words are often
> classic. Like beginning the word 'socks' with a 'c' instead of an 's.' Or
> her invention of a whole new and exciting ailment by changing the
> 'H' in Huntington's disease to a 'K.' 'Did I say it wrong?' she asks, as
> I dissolve in laughter. 'Tell me!' And I whisper it in her ear, and she
> guffaws. 'Let's try this word later,' advises Suzanne, knitting furiously.
> How can something so inherently frightening and frustrating be so
> hilarious. The only answer I can come up with is 'LAUREN!'"

As lively and loving as the portrayal was, I found it quite alarming. My dad was suggesting that all of my pre-stroke personality traits were still pronounced in me—I was opinionated, driven by humor, and very much in control. It was as if he had only seen what he had expected to see—or wanted to see. And I got the impression that his desire to entertain his readers was much stronger than his desire to inform them, and as a result, he had left me mistranslated. How could he not recognize the massive medical and linguistic changes I had gone through? Dramatic changes happen in everyone's lives, but mine took hold with no warning at all, most of them accomplished in a few seconds on a drenched bar floor. One minute I was singing along with a tune, and then blood was irrigating my head, flushing what I once thought of as my identity almost entirely away. Yes, I was revived. Yes, I was a girl again, with the same knuckles and same lips. But not the same girl. Dozens of similar e-mails appeared on the screen, but I was too overthrown to continue.

My father's portrait of me didn't match with the world I inhabited and didn't hint at the newfound Quiet, which had been at the very center of it for me.

In my journals, I wondered: Where did the girl from his letter end and the girl I was begin?

to tell dad off email
list
(for him)

dad to brings up to writing. he
writing. ~~bough~~ but my ~~experiences~~ story, I ~~g go~~ got him off
?
if was mine

I didn't immediately confront my father about what I had read in his e-mail outbox, partly because my mom told me he had stopped sending the notes out, and partly because, like many other incidents, I had mostly forgotten the whole thing. So when my dad invited me to join him on an errand at a Samy's Camera shop, I was more than happy to tag along.

As we walked down the printer aisle, my dad fiddled with the digital photo frames and vacuum-packed memory cards.

Been meaning to talk to you about something, he said. I've gotten so interested in all of this stuff you're going through. This whole language recovery. I guess it started when I was writing some little e-mails, but now I see something really coming together, thematically. Tinkering with the idea of writing about it with some more depth. Maybe even a boo—

You can't! I shouted at him. You won't! I was surprised by my own fervor, but I couldn't let him finish his sentence—certainly not with that word.

You cannot write about this. None of this. No more E-MAILS. NO BOOK. NOT *EVER*.

Was I making a scene? Or was the volume inside of me mainly produced by the blood trumpeting between my heart and throat?

How dare you? I hissed. This is not your life. This is mine.

All of the enthusiasm had drained from my dad's face, and when I heard his voice again it was kind and low.

Forgive me, honey, I'm just . . . Sorry. I didn't . . . I didn't even think. Of course.

Over the years, I know that conversations in my family sometimes leaned toward the argumentative. My father and I certainly had not been strangers to raised voices, but even in those moments, that tactic was part of productive debates. That day in Samy's Camera was different, though. I hadn't furthered a conversation; I had ended one. I had been curt to a man who had only ever been my advocate. What kind of stranger had I become?

Did I feel guilty when I confronted my father? Or did that come later, in retrospect? And if I had experienced a surge of pride about mobilizing the right language to stand up for myself, I can't exactly recall that. As the words had been pouring out of me in that moment, they had been as unwieldy and sticky as hot pitch, but they hardened into asphalt. Then there was a road before me. It had become something I could cross if I wanted to. This power of language had brought something into being. I was not yet certain how I could use language from this point on, or how on earth to use it to my advantage. I was only certain that I would not let anyone else speak for me.

PART THREE

INSTRUCTIONS

The Three Strangest Words

When I utter the word Future,
The first syllable is already headed for the past.

When I utter the word Silence,
I destroy it.

When I utter the word Nothing,
I create something no non-existence can contain.

WISŁAWA SZYMBORSKA

1

As part of our ongoing search for a speech and language pathologist, my mother called several nearby hospitals and universities, but with little success. Many practices weren't taking on new clients, others wouldn't take our insurance, and most of them had long waiting lists. I watched my mother's cheeks redden and tense every time she hung up the phone. She tried to shield her frustration from me, but after pursuing another lead that turned into a dead end, she hit her breaking point.

I keep hearing about this "critical period" you're in, she fumed. Aren't these people the experts? Don't they understand that you have to start therapy right away? It's like they would prefer you to have your speech therapy in a van on a street corner in Tijuana.

But in mid-October, we finally found Justine Sherman.

Justine had a private practice specializing in speech-language impairments. Her office was a converted home in Sierra Madre—ten minutes from my parents' house—with a small staff, mainly women. As she walked me through the building, I watched some of her other clients knock over blocks and plunge their fingers into one another's noses. I was the only patient there who wasn't a toddler.

Our first interview was in Justine's office. Her dark eyes shone from her slim face as she sat behind the desk in front of me.

Alicia is going to sit in on this consult, too, is that okay? she asked.

I looked over to the side of the room that was lined with bookshelves. A quiet girl near my age sat there and gave me a mild wave.

Sure, I said.

I know your case. Justine patted a thick folder on her desk. But I want you to tell me why *you* want to be in speech therapy. What is your biggest struggle these days?

Words, I guess. I forget words. Nouns, verbs—all kinds of words. I forget everything.

Justine started taking notes.

And reading, I added. I still have a lot of trouble reading, though I don't know why.

Justine's eyes bloomed. Tell me more about that.

I can just show you, I said, taking a paperback out of my purse. Soon after my release from the hospital in Edinburgh, Materson had given me his well-loved copy of John Grisham's *The Last Juror*.

I've been trying to read this book every day for a month, I explained, but I'm still not finished. It takes an hour for me to go through a paragraph, sometimes a full day to read a page. I don't even know what the book is about. What's the problem?

It's a good question, she said. The first thing I should tell you is that reading isn't just one thing. I am aware that you were a PhD student, so you might be especially interested in some of these mechanisms. There is a lexical issue to address, being exposed to a vocabulary you've forgotten. There are also syntactic issues, relating to the grammar of the sentence structures. Not to mention that prosody, the melody of sentences, is coming at you unevenly at this moment in time.

Lexical. Syntactic. Prosody. Justine wasn't dumbing things down for me, and I was grateful that she would engage with me at this level. The words were daunting, but somehow also familiar.

You have to organize all the information you are taking in, she said.

Then you have to visualize it. And then you have to remember everything you have just learned. Managing that convergence isn't at all simple. Quite the opposite.

I noticed myself relaxing into Justine's gentle authority.

Speaking, reading, and writing are related to one another, but they aren't the same thing, she explained. Language is a bit like a horse race. Any one of these capacities can leap ahead of the others for a bit. And while you are here, we'll work on all of these parts of your communication.

Over the next few days, Justine administered standardized tests to establish my current baseline. There were a number of questions I couldn't answer, and Justine's notes divided my word retrieval errors into categories: Semantic Locative, Semantic Coordinate, Semantic Associative, and Phonemic Omission.

For instance, I would say *orchestra* when I should have said *musician*, or *hoof* instead of *horseshoe*. These semantic errors were *locative* because I could isolate the *location* of the word I wanted to use, just not the exact term. Justine also noticed what Anne had mentioned two months earlier in Scotland: my oral-motor muscles wouldn't always coordinate into speech. Justine considered my apraxia mild at that point, though she noted: "Lauren has difficulty with multisyllabic words and often substitute(s) the vowel sounds." It was hard to make a distinction between voiced and unvoiced phonemes (*pop* versus *bop*), but Justine pointed out that I was usually aware when I was making those errors, a major improvement over Scotland. My irregular verbs continued to be problematic. I would say *swimmed* instead of *swam*, and couldn't identify the mistake. Justine wrote that my performance on memory tasks was "poor," and that I had "significant difficulty on the memory subset, which required [me] to remember both isolated and contextual information." She added: "[Lauren] appeared to perform better when contextual cues were provided rather than a straightforward assessment of her memory."

In spite of less-than-stellar performances on these tests, Justine was relatively positive about my case, writing that I was "a sharp, motivated woman with excellent potential." And I actually enjoyed taking the diagnostics because the existence of such tests was promising. It indicated that what had happened to me had happened before to someone else—to so many people, in fact, that a test had to be invented to evaluate all of them.

Justine promised that she and Alicia would have a syllabus prepared for me soon. As I was leaving after the final test, Justine plucked an armful of children's books from her stacks. They showed things in a house, things on a beach, things in an office.

These might help you remember everyday items when things slip your mind, she said. Don't stop reading your Grisham, though. It may seem a little weird to read *The Cat in the Hat* side by side with a thriller, but you might find they can actually complement each other.

When you can't find a word, it's like you are locked out of your own house. You check the windows to see if any of them are open. They aren't. You check the side doors to see if they were left ajar. But they are sealed shut. So you go under your house, squeezing through a crawl space, hoping to access the cellar that way. Since you can't go to the front door of your language, you *circumlocute.*

From Justine, I learned how to do that effectively.

How big is the thing you want to describe? What color is it? If it is an object, is it an item you use in your car? Is it something you wear? Something you eat? How does this thing feel in your hands?

During my endless circumlocutions, it often felt like I would say everything but the word itself. Justine told me not to get frustrated with this counterintuitive travel.

A lot of people with aphasia get themselves blocked, she said. When they can't say the perfect thing, they don't say anything at all. Don't do that to yourself. Pride can get in the way of recovery.

The way people learn and use language is often difficult to pin down. In spite of its ability to be honed in so many ways, it also comes to most people at the level of an instinct. As cognitive scientist and linguist Steven Pinker explains, "Language is a complex, specialized skill, which develops in the child spontaneously, without conscious effort or formal instruction, is deployed without awareness of its underlying logic. . . . Language is no more a cultural invention than is upright posture."

When I started speech therapy, I thought there would be a lot of linguistics involved in my treatment. I had some experience with that field, using some of its theories and models for papers in grad school. Since linguistics explores the way language functions, one would assume that it would be similarly involved in the way language malfunctions as well. But this is not the case. Language studies are hugely cross-disciplinary, spread among the therapeutic, academic, and scientific communities with no unifying theory shared among them. Experts in a single field often disagree with one another about how language affects cognition. And often, their studies didn't include people who have language disorders, only children learning language for the first time. So when a surgeon approaches a diseased heart, its well-known architecture guides his scalpel. But the anatomy of the "language organ" doesn't allow for such a simple approach. Hildred Schuell, a pioneer in aphasia research, points out that interventions in language disorders can be troubled from the very beginning of treatment because, "What you *do* about aphasia depends on what you think aphasia *is*."

Speech and Language Pathologists (SLPs) are at the front lines of this disorder. They are exposed to linguistic models as they go through their training and often rely on isolated linguistic tools to evaluate the deficits of their patients, like the diagnostic tests Justine gave me. But the work of the linguist is often theory driven, and that of the aphasiologist is much more research driven—it deals with the actual people in an actual room.

Aphasia can be easy to ignore or misdiagnose, especially in the older population it usually affects. If the patient doesn't respond well on language tests, that doesn't mean that language is the root of their problem. It could be their vision, their hearing, or the early signs of dementia. The approach of the SLP might look imprecise from the outside, but that's because it changes from patient to patient. It involves a certain amount of intuition. If music stimulates speech in a client, the therapist might start singing Christmas carols with them. If card games facilitate conversation and focused attention, they will play Go Fish during their sessions.

At some point in my development, I would become enthralled by the forensics of language again—its intricate maps and diagrams—though even now it's still hard for me to decode them. But Justine understood my interest early on. The way Justine picked up on my points of curiosity was her greatest strength, and allowing myself to remain curious proved to be my greatest asset.

2

San Diego was on fire. California had its earthquakes and mudslides, but it had its fires, too. It had full fire seasons, and this one was the biggest in the history of the county.

My mother called me from the office to alert me that her sister and her family had been evacuated from their home.

They're already en route to LA, she said. Can you clean up a bit?

When I went outside, the weather was postcard worthy, with no sign of the fires raging two hours south. Soon, though, my extended family arrived in two cars, each filled with bags overstuffed with clothing and toiletries. Jewelry boxes were left open on the seats. The large, sepia family portraits that usually hung throughout their home were wrapped in dark blankets. Even with all this, they almost immediately began second-guessing what they had taken and what they had left behind. I hadn't experienced this kind of rearview reflection after leaving New York; it had been more than a month since I'd left and I still couldn't think of anything I missed.

Once they had emptied the cars and gotten the kids settled, my uncle and aunt beelined for the electrical outlets to plug in and turn on their minute-to-minute reports of the fire's path. I ducked outside to escape the hubbub, and as always, I had my journal in hand.

Before long, my eight-year-old cousin, Elle, caught sight of me and scurried across the lawn in my direction.

Found you! she said, giggling, wrapping her impish body around me. We were the only female grandchildren in this family, almost twenty years apart and rarely in the same place, but she loved doing all sorts of projects with me. What she couldn't possibly understand was that circumstances were different now, especially when it came to language.

You wanna help me out with something, Cousin Lauren?

I guess that depends, I said cautiously. What's the assignment?

Reading aloud, she said. We take turns. I read a page, and then you read the next.

Well . . . I said, looking down to her young, eager eyes. We might as well try.

We started to pass her book back and forth, both attempting to voice the words before us, but achieving anything that resembled an easy tempo was difficult. Suddenly, a bizarre fact became startlingly clear to me: my eight-year-old cousin and I were at the same reading level.

On one of her pages, Elle got stuck on the word *tarantula*, and though I tried to correct her, the word proved impossible for me too.

Tarantella? I tried. Tam-tat-tar . . .

Annoyed, I heard myself stuttering like a car engine until the word finally rattled off my tongue correctly: *Tarantula!* I said with triumph.

What is it? Elle asked me. This Sir Spatula?

I linked my hands together and I lunged at her, as if my fingers were spider legs.

This is a *tarantula!*

Gleefully dodging my tickles, Elle rolled down to the grass, where she found my pen and journal.

I have another idea! Elle said. Do you think we can write a story together?

Sure thing. I grabbed the pen from her. You first, kiddo.

This is a story that is not about my brain, she began. It is about Elle's brain.

I stopped transcribing. What did Elle know about the aneurysm? What had she been told? At her age, it couldn't have been much. But she might have overheard some phone conversations, detected whispered concerns, picked up some key words. Elle was thinking about brains, but she had cast herself as the main character in that story, instead of me.

Keep going, I told her. You tell me what happens and I'll just write it down.

Elle invented a fable about a girl named Elle. This girl had an impressive brain until the day it fell off her body. She grew a new brain, and this one (my cousin emphasized) was humungous. But it failed her too. The Elle from the story continued to grow, and lose, these disposable brains. I loved the twists in Elle's storytelling. Only after the girl actually died and became a ghost did she acquire her Happily Ever After.

When we finished, Elle snatched the journal from me, and looked at our combined effort. She flashed me a grin, displaying both the gaps in her mouth and her teeth in progress. Then she darted off, eager to share her story.

Elle and her family spent less than a week in Los Angeles before the fires were contained and they were given the all clear to return home. After seeing everyone off at the base of the driveway, Gram asked me to come inside her cottage and sit with her as she finished her coffee.

A year of close calls, she said, rapping her arthritic fingers on her round wooden table. Wouldn't you say?

I told her I wasn't quite sure what she meant.

My grandmother listed a few things. There was the San Diego fire, which had spared our family's lives and home. There was my cousin Spencer, whose major motorbike accident a month before my own injury had crushed parts of his spine, but to everyone's relief, he had not been left paralyzed.

And, of course, there is your aneurysm, my grandma said. Wouldn't you consider your own medical emergency a "close call"?

Oh, I said. Yeah, I guess.

Interesting, my grandmother said. You remember when I worked in the hospital, don't you?

I nodded. As a child, I used to visit her at work. She was the most senior nurse on the ward, and almost everyone answered to her.

Well, I did a lot of things in that place, even though it was in a somewhat isolated corner of Northeast Montana, she said. I managed patients with all sorts of injuries, delivered babies, and personally helped set up the Glasgow medical airlift and doctors' exchange. I was real proud of that. But in those five decades, I was never able to save anyone who had an aneurysm rupture.

Oh no? I asked. Why not?

Sometimes I wonder if you really understand what happened to you, Lauren. A rupture is often a death sentence, and treatment has everything to do with location. Though I saw about a dozen cases like yours, everyone from our little hospital died in transport to somewhere else.

Gram took another sip of her black coffee.

You've got a very serious thing up there in your noggin, she said. The sort of thing only a specialist can treat, and only a few places in the world can do that well. After an aneurysm's rupture, everything needs to be aligned perfectly for a patient's survival. I thank God you had all the resources you needed to be able to get through this and I count my blessings every day.

My grandmother had always been a church-going woman, and though I had been interested in religion, and even studied it academically for years, I didn't practice formally before or after the rupture. I was relieved that Gram hadn't assumed that my near-death experience had been a religious one. There had never been tunnels of light or out-of-body experiences. Once the hemorrhage began, I had no clear memories until after the surgery was finished, and I certainly hadn't woken up from this procedure thinking I should be a better Catholic.

But there had been the Quiet. I had been exposed to this incredible sense of order, and it had been so pervasive, so all-encompassing, I felt its traces in me could never really disappear. I was immensely grateful for this experience, which had altered the attention I paid to the world. In fact, *grateful* was too small a word.

Don't you ever forget how lucky you are, my grandmother said. Because you happened to be at the *right* place, at the *right* time.

And on this point, my grandmother and I were in complete agreement.

3

One crisp fall morning, I joined my parents on their walk before work. I did this fairly often, but it was getting harder and harder to get up this early because my dark bedroom didn't take in much light at all. Before I had left for college years ago, I had given the space a moody teenager paint job, a blue that was almost black.

I think it might be time for a change, I said to my mother.

Finally, my mom said. Been counting the days till you'd outgrow that gloom. She pointed out the pumpkins on neighbors' porches and changing leaves on the trees around us. Would you consider something autumnal? she asked.

A vivid image came to mind. Right before Edinburgh, I had been in Paris. I had been awed by the way light struck the weathered facades there. At dawn and dusk, the French walls glowed like embers.

What about red? I said. Wouldn't it be great to have a red room?

Mom had been leading the brisk pace of the walk, but her sneakers squeaked on the curb as she halted abruptly.

You can't be serious, she said. Lauren, are you really suggesting we should just go from midnight blue to blood red?

No, I corrected her. *Parisian* red.

. . .

Why do I remember Paris in the way I do? When I think of Paris I always think of it with Edinburgh—a bound pair, like chicken and rice or balloons and birthday parties. And in the months since the rupture, Paris had been just as important a place as Edinburgh. It was a touchstone, and unlike other things in my life, something I remembered somewhat clearly.

I had arrived in France a week before I was due to meet BJ and Laura in Scotland. Of course I remember Paris, because this was my first trip to the city, and it had broken up my otherwise predictable New York routine. But much more than that, I think I remember Paris because of the girl I had been there—this was the version of myself that everyone seemed to remember. Unfractured. Before the fall. That was someone of whom I was trying to get glimpses of. In France, I had stayed with my friend and former professor Michael Krass, whom I had known for years. He was like an uncle to me. The cool kind of uncle with whom you can speak freely, who spoils you a bit, and gives you more freedom than you have at home. He was a successful costume designer in Manhattan and had rented a great apartment for the summer in the middle of Paris—two floors, with a whole guest suite to itself on the lower level. In certain contexts, it might have been considered inappropriate for a male professor to offer a room to his female student, but his invitation couldn't have been any more platonic. In our long friendship, his exclusive preference for male partners had never been a secret.

Just come to France, he said. The only reason to rent an apartment in Paris is to have visitors. And you can stay for a whole month before you head out to Edinburgh, if you want to. . . .

Though my financial constraints were substantial, I was not going to say no to the offer. I could stay for a week, at least. Krass's apartment was situated on the appealing Isle St. Louis, only two blocks away from the short footbridge that led to Notre Dame. Krass showed me the trick of unlocking his bright violet door, and he handed me my own set of keys.

To come and go as you please, he said. And if you want to bring back an overnight guest, I'll be the soul of discretion. He winked, and led me up to the roof deck.

From the private terrace, four flights above the street, we could look down and watch the bustle below, the air saturated with the honey and butter wafting up from the bakery on the ground floor. In front of us was the magnificent cathedral, its buttresses resembling a tremendous rib cage. We looked up to the transit of clouds, and for a few moments, near dawn and dusk, every cream-colored building glowed this singular shade of red.

Living in a space that could always capture the light show of sunrise and sunset was ideal. And if I was going to be in California for a while, that was the kind of thing I wanted to re-create in my bedroom.

4

Per Dr. Russin's recommendation, my mother finally got me an appointment at USC, with Dr. George Teitelbaum, director of interventional neuroradiology. As I sat in the waiting room, I filled out the requisite paperwork with my mother's help. On top, she noted the date: October 30, 2007.

There weren't many introductions, and once I met Dr. Teitelbaum, he commenced with my exam. He asked me to touch my nose with my finger, first with my eyes open, then with my eyes closed. Next he wanted me to balance on one leg. Could I feel it when he stroked my arm? What about there? He gave me the name of three items in the room (*pen, clock, coat*), and five minutes later asked if I remembered them by name.

I completed the tasks as instructed, but without much enthusiasm. I assumed this would be the first and only time Dr. Teitelbaum and I would ever meet. This was just procedure. The plan was for Dr. Teitelbaum to write up a report of our meeting and send it along to Dr. Russin's office. I didn't know at the time that my doctors sent reports back and forth to each other, and it would be a while before I realized that patients could request such documents for themselves.

When I eventually saw Dr. Teitelbaum's report, it was hard for me to read, partially because of my aphasia, but also because of the pervasive medical terminology. I would review this report time and again, over a period of several years. And as my knowledge base grew, it was like reading a new document every time.

"Thank you for allowing me to consult on your patient, Lauren Marks, a very pleasant 27-year-old female that on August 24, 2007, suffered a subarachnoid hemorrhage due to a large left middle cerebral trifurcation that was treated in Edinborough (sic), Scotland . . . satisfactorily occluded with the use of bare platinum and HydroCoils."

Very pleasant. It was a compliment, so I probably noticed that early in my first read. *Satisfactorily* was good—I knew that immediately. But *occluded* sounded bad. The term meant *blocked.* However, this block was the dam that kept blood from refilling the aneurysm, so occluded was positive, in this case. And *platinum* and *HydroCoils* made me sound bionic. People who stole copper from street lamps would plunder my skull if they only knew.

Buried mid-paragraph on the second page, there were a couple of sentences that included a word I had never heard before: *recanalization.* Did it have something to do with canals? Assuming it was just another complicated term that dealt with some minute detail about my case, I only glanced at this passage.

"I would recommend that she undergo a follow-up angiogram at 6 months' time," Dr. Teitelbaum advised. He reported that he had gone through my tests from Scotland and noted that the "aneurysm appeared to be well treated by coil embolization."

"However," he continued, "I would estimate that the chance of recanalization of such a large aneurysm is fifteen to twenty percent."

The odds appeared to be very much in my favor here, but this was something I really should have looked up sooner.

5

Don't burn your bridges. A stitch in time saves nine. Today's lesson was on idioms, and Alicia wanted me to translate the phrases, to explain what they meant and why people used them. It shouldn't have been too difficult since I had heard and used them throughout my life. But the sayings didn't stick in my head the same way anymore, didn't click against my teeth the way they should have. The table we were working at was filled with colorful puzzles, games, and dry erase boards. We sat in plastic chairs, low to the ground.

It was becoming increasingly clear that I had retained only a vague aptitude for these sorts of phrases. I usually knew what people meant when they used them, but mainly from evaluating a person's tone or body language. I couldn't produce them on my own, couldn't repeat them back if I was asked to. It wasn't that my aphasia made me too literal—I understood that language could be figurative—but why these words? Why in this order? Idioms tended to be loaded with images, which would put my brain into overdrive; it was hard to keep my attention focused on Alicia when *flying off the handle* conjured up soup pots sprouting pigeon wings.

I feel like a million bucks, Alicia said to me. What do you think that means, Lauren?

It means I am . . . happy, I said. It means that bucks, which is money, is like happiness.

Basically, yeah, she said. It's an analogy. We're going to work on analogies more next week, she added as she flipped through her pile of worksheets, ready to tackle another subject.

Wait, I said. Go back.

I wanted Alicia to explain. It sounded to me that the phrase suggested that money had feelings, and we should feel the same way money does. Or maybe money was something you should feel on your skin. Or maybe you could buy a lot of things with a million bucks, and those things would make you feel happy. But none of these options resonated with me. A million of anything was far too much. It was like watching a cell divide and multiply in front of me, the mutation occurring more quickly than I could track.

I knotted my fingers inside the pockets of my dress, grinding my teeth. I pressed Alicia on this: Why would we want to feel like a million bucks?

Don't think I follow, Lauren, she said. Can you explain your issue?

The idiom itself was the issue. It seemed to be about greed. And for a culture to understand these words implicitly, it meant that this truth had been widely assimilated.

Facing the music was equally complex. It meant to be held accountable for something, but in my mind, the words were too animated. When I closed my eyes, I'd see a jazz funeral marching down a street in New Orleans, musicians surrounding an open casket with their blaring brass sounding into a cold, unhearing ear. The man in the box was *facing* his music.

If this exercise is upsetting you, Alicia said, we don't have to keep doing it.

Before the rupture my face was easy to read, but it was even more so after it. I couldn't disguise my distress, but Alicia had overestimated the gravity of the situation. I didn't want to stop working on idioms. In fact, I wanted more of them. I was starting to crave their challenge. An idiom was a parable. It was like a covenant between the words and those who received the words. With them, I was observing how words could twist and plunge, reference and implicate, echo and haunt. I grasped ideas faster than I would have if I had been a child because of the isolated pockets of preserved knowledge and experience present from before the rupture. But any deftness I might have had coexisted with many other rudimentary linguistic difficulties. Odd as it might sound, aphasia gave me an opportunity to re-encounter the enthusiasm for language I had felt when growing up. After the stroke, I was manifesting a host of disfluent symptoms that often made me dependent on those around me. But when I approached words now, it was with reverence again, an easy sense of awe. Recommitting myself to the contract of language was thrilling, but it also made me a tourist in my native tongue.

Justine and I were in the private office where she conducted my sessions. As always, she was eager to hear about my ideas regarding the next steps in my therapy.

I want to try to do an essay or something, I said. Not just fiddle in my journals.

You don't think you are able to start something like that yourself? Justine asked.

Not really, I admitted. When I was a PhD student, I wrote essays as easily as I made oatmeal. Now I don't even know how to start one.

What do you think is stopping you? she asked.

I tried to explain that in the past, ideas fell into place naturally on the page. A thought in one sentence would effortlessly develop into the next sentence as a gentle stream of consciousness. But now, it took so long to write a full sentence that by the time I finished it I had forgotten whatever other ideas I might have had. The traffic jam became a desert highway.

Justine made a radical suggestion: give up the way I used to write. When a topic came up now, I should jot down all the words that it would call to mind. Names of people, places, things. I shouldn't try to put it into a structure immediately. Who cared if I wrote a bad sentence? Putting the ideas down was the most important part, and making the piece sound good could come later. The approach was feasible, and I was overjoyed she had come up with it. The next week, she brought in a writing assignment for me on the subject of "perseverance."

You don't have to finish this quickly, she said. We can take as long as we want.

The prompt page had quotations from Nelson Mandela, Ghandi, and Helen Keller. For inspiration, she explained. Some people who've triumphed in the face of adversity.

I glanced at the page, but there was something about the idea that troubled me.

What about . . . ummm . . . Obben . . . you know. Scientist. New Mexico . . . I showed her with my hands. BOOM.

Oppenheimer? she asked.

Yeah, I said. That's it.

Umm. She paused. You want to make J. Robert Oppenheimer the subject of your perseverance essay?

No, no, that is not what I meant. I slowly explained to Justine that on the way into therapy that day, a radio segment had been discussing the *Enola Gay*, the plane that dropped the bomb on Hiroshima. Like all the other figures on Justine's prompt, Oppenheimer had done something the world had never seen before, in a time of great adversity. She was careful not to interrupt me as I tried to cobble my reasoning together.

That's true, she said, her tone still a little uneasy.

Well? I asked her. See how that turned out? Perseverance is not always a good thing.

Justine broke into a laugh.

Had no idea where you were going with that! she exclaimed. But it's an astute observation to make: the unintentional consequences of perseverance. Lauren, I think you've found yourself a theme.

The assignments from speech therapy had gotten me motivated, and I wanted to find sources to explore the subjects of perseverance and idioms. But to do that, I would need my mother to drive me to a bookstore.

Bookstores had been a touchy subject in my family, namely because of my brief stint working at The Strand years earlier. I'd been hired my sophomore year at NYU and convinced my parents the job was ideal for me: not only would I be gainfully employed, but I'd also be getting steep discounts on books I would be buying anyway.

Summer at The Strand. For The Girl I Used to Be it had been pure bliss. At the time, I lived on the same block where a young Allen Ginsberg had written "Kaddish." On the way to work, I'd pass St. Mark's Church, where I heard an elderly Lawrence Ferlinghetti read some of his new poems. During my shift at the store, I'd park myself on top of ladders to look like I was working, but usually I was just reading. In a place like The Strand, with its stacks and sheer volume of books, you rarely found what you were looking for, but often a better treasure would present itself. And while I was discovering Kundera, Szymborska, Miłosz, I was also falling in love for the first time.

Jason was another acting student at NYU; his frame was thin but athletic and his delicate dark features showcased the very best of his Chinese and European ancestry. He was impulsive, sometimes reckless, and considered himself a hopeless romantic. He loved to surprise me at work. I'd be crouching down to replace items near the warped floorboards, and I would suddenly feel his small hands clasped around my hips. There was no air-conditioning, so the ceiling fans would circulate the assortment of odors: the damp in the old books, the fresh glue bindings in the new ones, the sweat and car exhaust clinging to the glistening summer bodies. The Strand never felt like a public place to me. It was like a church, but when Jason and I managed our furtive embraces, I was certain all of the saints on the shelves encouraged our behavior. I was rich in words, rich in love. A fall from that grace was hard to imagine.

But after only a few months, I had to quit the position. All the money that should have gone to groceries and rent was instead going to new book purchases. My mother and father were frustrated when I asked them to help me out, and it became an established family fact that I couldn't be relied upon to exert common financial sense where books were concerned.

I don't think I remembered this detailed interpersonal history when I asked my mother to take me to Vroman's Bookstore in Pasadena that November afternoon. But I did have an indistinct impression that places like this were off-limits for me somehow. When I brought up this sinking sensation to my mother, she reminded me of some of the conversations we had over the years about not spending too much money in bookstores. However, she was quick to add that after my rupture and diagnosis, she had started to worry I'd never want to set foot in a bookstore again and was happy that she'd been wrong.

I think this field trip is long overdue, she said with a smile.

Though I loved Vroman's as much as I loved The Strand, I'd loved the former for much longer. When I was a kid, my parents' first office together was on the same street as the independent shop, making the bookstore feel a bit like the extension of our own family library. This time, Mom left me in the nonfiction stacks, near the cookbooks and the metal tree of hanging aprons. As I stood among the shelves again, I realized not much had changed. It still brought on a sense of peace.

When I found a book on English phrases, I quickly turned to the index and stumbled upon a short entry for *facing the music*. There were a number of speculations about how the phrase came to be, beginning with the military. In the American army, when a soldier was dishonorably discharged, a drummer played while he was marched out of the barracks. This was the "music" of his forced exit. The second provenance was theatrical. In a classic proscenium theater, there was a stage, an orchestra pit, and the audience. Since, architecturally speaking, the orchestra is situated between the performer and the audience, the actress was always facing her music. I kept flipping between the index and other expressions, trying to learn as much as possible. This was exactly what I'd needed.

My mother saw my enthusiasm and bought the book for me on the spot. Not only was it interesting, it was also on my reading level. My memory couldn't accommodate a long or complicated story and I was unable to manage multiple narrative threads. But in this book, each saying had a completely self-contained entry and was rarely longer than a paragraph or two. This turned out to be the perfect length if I wanted to both learn new information and retain it.

I started to make a game of the index. First, I'd guess the origin of the idiom, giving it an imagined biography. Then, I would read the actual story about how it came into use. It was like a makeshift version of the game Balderdash. BJ and Laura never exactly warmed to it, but I could usually enlist Jonah to play it when he called. And my friend Grace enjoyed the game most of all. Having met at an all-girls high school, we had read the same books, written the same assignments, grown up in language together. Now this wordy practice was something we could do together again.

Guess how this phrase started! I'd say. *I'll scratch your back if you scratch mine.*

Our guesses were consistently incorrect, but it was still a valuable exercise. These origin stories were vividly drawn. They were alive with images, so I could find a reason for why each word was used the way it was. I still wasn't able to memorize the phrases very well, but I started to hear their melody a bit more.

Facing the Music was the jazz funeral. And the army barracks. And the actress onstage. Because a story gave an idiom a life, and three stories would make that life more diverse.

6

She wanted to discuss our plan (maps). What we will do. What my "goal,"
my end result from therapy. ~~What it means~~ *I take from her questions* ~~are~~
~~what I will be~~ *that she wants me to describe what will be called recovery.*
But this is more complicated than she suggests. Heal the wound. Scar. I
try to ~~complicate~~ *trouble the question.* ~~For~~ *There is no "back" or "retreat" or*
"recover." There is only cover. Advance. Forward. What she calls recovery
sounds like life before and that is not on my map.

Alicia and I were in a room that smelled of bubblegum and sunscreen at
the back of the therapy complex. I no longer had the hesitation I had come
into the building with weeks ago. In fact, I was here so often I was starting
to develop a newfound confidence.

So how long do we get to do these sessions? I asked Alicia. A few more
weeks? A couple of months? When do we stop?

Alicia's voice became hesitant, and her right hand wandered to her
head, uncomfortably resting on a few loose strands of hair near her
shoulder.

Aphasia is . . . well, aphasia is not something that can be exactly cured.

Has Justine talked to you about that? We are here to help you build some compensatory strategies to make it easier for you to communicate.

I understand. And I want to stay here as long as I can. But you said I'm getting better much faster than you expected, right?

That's right, she said, and started to unconsciously tug at that unruly patch of hair.

Yeah, I think I'm doing really well, I said. I am feeling pretty confident with my words.

Tug. tug. And that's . . . good, Alicia said, tugging a little more firmly now. That's sort of . . . the point. *Tug.*

I felt I had to put her at ease. Speech therapy is the best part of my week, I said, trying to lighten the mood. I'm just asking—when do I have to stop? And what am I supposed to do next?

Well, this might be a good time to define some goals for yourself in therapy. Alicia seemed to give up on her mission to tug and smooth her hair into submission, and finally let her eyes rest on me. Do you know what you'd like your recovery to look like? Because it probably won't be exactly like what your life was before.

Like most people I'd interacted with since the stroke, Alicia was assuming I wanted my life to look the same way. But that wasn't something I was yearning for. For example, my brother was going to be in town again soon, and I was looking forward to engaging with him in person. Over the occasional phone call, I sensed our dynamic wasn't the same as before, but that wasn't so bad, was it? I wasn't trying to get back to the life before. How could I make Alicia understand?

This wasn't a retreat. This was an advance.

7

When you <u>acclimate</u> (?) in your environment, the environment
dissappears. ~~The~~ As quickly as you recognize your present, your past erases.

My past is erasing even as I ~~re~~ teaching/practing myself words like
"erasing" and "practing." After each syllabul repairs, it is forgotten.

–Dread has returned. Not as thorny as it was. My own memories arise
fear I don't know. Now death is plausible and now (terrifying)? not
terrifying. but something else. dreddful?

<u>Sp. Therapy</u> Isn't just communicate/ing. It takeing on a world of thoughts
many occupied with anxiety and fears.

There was so much I enjoyed about speech therapy, but I was also becoming
aware that my rehabilitation was just as much about input as it was about
output. Communication, to me, now meant more than just being able to
create sentences and say words; it entailed taking in the world of thoughts
and ideas of those around me, and some of those thoughts produced anxiety.

I thought back to that day in Edinburgh when Jonah and I had talked about death in the Patersons' garden. What had changed in the span of two months? I knew something had.

Day by day, my vocabulary was steadily building. In Los Angeles, I was joyously reacquainting myself with positive terms like *recovery*, *better*, and *healthy*. I loved the specificity I was becoming able to employ. But soon, these words would be paired with others, and their antonyms were thornier and much less welcome, words like *sickness*, *morbidity*, and *permanent*. Because when a mind grasps a semantic concept like *fragile*, it is bound to reflect on its opposite at some point.

Am I fragile? Am I likely to break?

It is incredibly difficult to understand how information is stored in our brain, and what form our knowledge takes there. A popular view in psycholinguistics is that the human mind groups associated ideas, represented in words, in what is called a "semantic network." In this weblike arrangement, closely related concepts, like categories and attributes, appear very near one another spatially as *nodes*. Less-associated concepts have more distance between their nodes.

This idea of the *semantic network* resonated with me, and matched my experience quite closely. Instead of a web, however, I envisioned it as a tree. If I were to create one of these personal charts now, it would begin with the trunk of that tree. For this exercise, I'll chart a network for the word *blue*.

There would be branches on this tree, bearing fruit representing other colors like *green*, *orange*, and *yellow*. Another set of branches would represent aspects of the natural world that I associate with blueness, like *sky*, *sea*, and *river*. Other branches would represent cultural touchstones: songs, paintings, and plays that mentally linked with blueness. But once the rupture occurred, this scene changed dramatically. Aphasia was like a mad gardener that sliced the branches and limbs away from the trunk. This sparse topiary cut me off from my usual points of reference, keeping me from associating my thoughts with one another, and affecting the predilections and predictions inside my mind.

Before the stroke, *blue* might have brought to mind Picasso's blue period. That could get me thinking about the Picasso exhibit that was on in Edinburgh at the same time as the Fringe Festival. From there, I could think about my eighth-grade art class where I originally learned about Picasso. I could think of my ostrich-necked teacher with her big glasses on their long, colorfully beaded chain. There might even be the distant yearning for her to turn around and praise my sketches, or the fearful excitement for the boy I had a crush on to glance over in my direction.

After the stroke, one thought could not lead to another in this way, which made me feel like a stranger in the forest of my own memories. Language is at its best in its firmness—in its ability to make ephemeral things more like objects. And although not all thoughts are paired with language, thoughts without language tend to be much more fleeting. Things were starting to change during speech therapy, as I was reattaching the branches to the trees of my language. But ultimately, this process of reconnection would take many years and my perception was shifting constantly. It was not the formal end of the Quiet by any means, but my self-directed speech was starting to resurface. I had enough language to view, analyze, and describe myself differently. Where there had once been vacancy, there was now clutter.

When I had spoken to Jonah in that garden in Edinburgh, telling him I wasn't afraid to die, it might have been easier to say it, easier even to think it, without the cluster of associations I had spent a lifetime amassing. The mainly negative thoughts (or at least the ones that were represented in language) that were related to death and dying in my mind just weren't as present to me at all.

It's interesting that my first moments of nagging fear were not when I was facing a lack of language, but when I began to regain it. The process was introducing a number of new variables, an abundance that I wasn't yet able to sift through or organize. This lack of clarity makes it difficult to pinpoint exactly when my inner voice finally turned on, and what form it took when it did, though I suspect my uneasiness in November was at least partially related to its re-engagement. The Quiet was no longer my default, or at least not always. It was like something in the air just wasn't quite right.

8

It's your brother's twenty-first birthday today, my dad said, while preparing his morning coffee. He was speaking to me between the pulses of the grinding beans. *Grind, grind, stop.* It's a major rite of passage. *Grind, grind, stop.* And he isn't going to want to go out with his old fogey parents. *Grind, grind, stop.* I wonder if you might consider taking him out tonight, if you feel up to it.

I considered the idea. I guess I can manage it, as long as I nap beforehand.

Attagirl, my dad said, patting me on the shoulder. Mike's lucky to have an older sister like you. I remember how you used to climb into his crib with him. Even though you two are almost seven years apart, you were such a slip of a girl, you really could fit in there fine. If he had been crying for a while, you'd try to help calm him down. You've always been looking after him, and even though he doesn't say it, Mike still looks up to you.

I wasn't sure how to respond to that. I appreciated the praise but felt a little ambivalent about it, especially since my memories weren't nearly as sharp as my dad's. And things had been a little off with Michael since he'd arrived home from Monterey. His first day back, he'd found me in my bedroom ripping up carpet, surrounded by cans of red paint.

That's quite a mess, he said, looking around. I wasn't in my bedroom proper—it was all wood floors in there—the carpeted area was more like an anteroom on the way to the bathroom. Mike and I shared that bathroom, a kind of Jack and Jill setup, with the toilet and shower in the shared space, but the two sinks were on our opposing sides. This is a lot of change to take in, he remarked, sounding a bit uneasy. You aren't planning to tear up my side too, are you?

I shot him a weary grin. You're safe, I said. The mess stays on my side. I was dizzy from the astringent smell of adhesive remover. We had spoken over the phone a few times since Scotland, but hadn't seen each other since my return to LA. As my brother helped me stumble to my feet, we kept holding on to each other, in a tight hug.

After a moment or two, he fumbled through his jeans, producing a tiny green bag of pot. He shot me a playful grin. His skin was so light that even this blush of pink made his cheeks look as red as his hair.

Want to join me downstairs? he asked. About to roll one.

I declined. There was a period of time when I would've enjoyed a smoke with my brother, but it was difficult enough to get through a regular day without adding the obstacle of intoxication. My mind was pre-scrambled.

Suit yourself. He shrugged. But you are missing out—this is primo Northern California bud.

We can talk without smoking, can't we? I asked. There was so much Mike didn't know about what had happened in Scotland or what it was like being back in LA after a decade away from the family home. This room renovation was the least important of it all. When he had called, he was never really calling for me, and we didn't chat long. He had always been interested in my life; we used to talk openly and often, though as the older sister I had given more advice than I received. Now, face-to-face, I assumed he might have a couple of questions for me, and I wanted to give him an opportunity to address topics he might have been too nervous to ask about earlier.

We can talk about the aneurysm, if you want, I said. It doesn't make me feel uncomfortable.

Oh, well . . . Mike looked down to his faded black Converse sneakers. Not right now, he said. Just really glad you're home.

And that was it. Our conversations hadn't really evolved since then.

Late that night, we walked over to The Rancho, a local dive bar known for its pool table, jukebox, and stale pretzels. Mike ordered a bottle of Heineken and a Maker's Mark. I got a Diet Coke. For years, whiskey had been my drink of choice as well, but I had preferred Wild Turkey with maraschino cherries instead of ice. I had a poet-bartender friend back in New York who had dubbed the combination "the Dorothy Parker," for the girls who looked like girls but drank like boys. Since it was my signature drink, my pal would sling it as soon as he saw me walking up to the door of his pub and have it waiting for me before I even sat down. But I hadn't had alcohol, or even a cup of coffee, since my time in Edinburgh. Now that I was starting to actually hear my language hiccups, I was getting the impression that to the outside world I sounded drunk even when I was sober. The bartender passed Mike's beer to him but I cupped my hand over my brother's glass before he poured the whiskey.

Forgetting something? I glared at the bartender.

But he did not receive my meaning. Mike stepped in to translate.

What my sister is trying to say is that she would like you to card me. Mike popped his wallet open. But I've been legal for eleven minutes now. See?

Unimpressed, the bartender nodded at him, and silently poured the rest of his order.

I nursed my Coke, my elbow stuck in some kind of syrupy residue on the worn bar. Mike rambled a little about his film classes as he drank, but he mainly talked about his ongoing difficulties with his girlfriend, Amber. I didn't know her personally—she had not been around before I moved to New York—but I had seen pictures of her on my brother's cell phone. She was striking. Her curtain of long, dark hair emphasized her light eyes, and though she wasn't very tall, she was slim, and could easily have been mistaken for a model. But my folks had long suspected that she might have some substance abuse problems, and the more Mike talked about her, the more it sounded like these issues may well have been inherited. My brother said that Amber's dad was in and out of rehab and he hinted her mother would occasionally take Amber's prescriptions recreationally. Mike and I had kept an open conversation about drug use over the years. I knew he drank, had taken mushrooms in college, and smoked pot (he and I had shared a couple of joints over the years). But he had a full-blown anxiety about synthetic drugs, which mostly kept him away from the hard stuff. I was fully aware that his moderation was mild in comparison to my own college years in New York, or my parents' hippie days in Berlin.

Mike said things were at a low point with him and Amber. He wasn't sure what he should do. I registered what Mike was saying, but I didn't comment on it and didn't really think I had to. My dad had called this birthday drink a "rite of passage," and I thought that getting Mike tipsy was the extent of my duties. Giving relationship advice was not in my job description for the night.

My brother and I didn't stay at the bar long, and afterward, we did the ten-minute walk home, arm in arm.

The phone in the garage apartment rang a little after 4:00 a.m., jolting me awake. It took me a moment to remember where I was. I had been sleeping in the back house because the paint was drying in my bedroom in the main house. The phone kept ringing. I didn't pick up the call; at that hour, it had to have been a wrong number. Suddenly, there were footsteps on my stairs, the apartment door swung open, and my mother appeared in the dark.

Hide these! she said, tossing something small and metallic at me. And then she was gone.

I turned on the light and saw my brother's car keys at the end of my bed. Perplexed but obedient, I buried them inside my underwear drawer. Then I felt the floor of my apartment shaking: the garage door was opening. I got out of bed and looked out the windows that faced the main house. The sky was dark, but all the lights were on in there. My mother had pulled the car out into the driveway. Amber was in the front passenger seat. But I couldn't figure out why she was there, or why she looked furious.

Mike had now appeared at the back door, pleading with my mother.

Stop, he said. You are ripping my love away from me!

Not in my house, she snapped. Never in my house.

And with that, my mother pushed past him and drove off, taking Amber home, even though she lived two hours north of us.

By the time I stumbled down into the main house, my brother was gone. The only indication he had been there was the empty handle of Smirnoff left open on the kitchen table.

My father told me that he and my mom had woken up to raised voices in the bedroom next to theirs, and felt the plaster wall buzzing as things were hurled against it. Mike and Amber were fighting—and it was a huge one. They had been smoking and drinking all night and when my parents came in, they were physically clawing at each other. My parents had to pry them apart. The whole scene my dad was describing was hard for me to imagine—Mike and my dad had always had hot tempers, but that had never manifested in bodily harm in our household, not by a mile. I stood there in shock.

I then became desperate to find Mike, needing him to make sense of it all. When I was actually in the room with him a few minutes later, I was still dumbstruck. I was a transparent moth and he was the irresistible porch light. As a ghost-bug without a mouth, I silently flitted around him as he went into the downstairs closet, the laundry room, the basement. If I could have spoken, I would have asked: *What is happening? What are you doing? Are you okay?* But my bug-brain and bug-mouth just wouldn't connect.

Mike weakly shambled around, winded, spent, and drunk. While Dad cleaned up the mess Mike and Amber had made around the house, I managed to get Mike to his bedroom. He climbed into his twin bed, and I lay down in the one beside him. He passed out almost immediately. As I lay across from him, I wondered how I had missed this storm brewing. I realized that my focus had been on myself since my return to Los Angeles. I'd been occupied by the sensation of being a brand-new person. But for the very first time, it hit me that this could be problematic for others in ways I had not anticipated. There was a world outside of me, populated with people I knew. And some of these people might still need things from me. The old me. I thought back to my dad's statement about how Mike was lucky to have an older sister like me. But there was no doubt in my mind that I had looked after him much better before the rupture. Things were different now. What should—or could—a good older sister do?

If I had been following my usual script with Mike, after he had taken his turn bemoaning the woes of his relationship back at the bar, I would have shared my own experiences with him, letting him know that we had a lot in common. My twenty-first birthday had also been ruined by a relationship going sour.

The breakup with Jason had been a messy one. We had been together just shy of two years when he initiated our split, but neither of us could exactly commit to breaking up. So I left town that summer to work for a theater festival in Williamstown, Massachusetts, mainly to avoid him. After I'd left, though, he'd call me in moments of drunken regret to tell me that he had just slept with some girl or another, then apologize for being an idiot, and go on about how he knew I was the love of his life and the future mother of his children. Almost every phone call with him left me miserable. I wouldn't have invited him to my twenty-first birthday, a date that fell while I was out of town, but I was intensely relieved when he showed up. Unsurprisingly, though, the heartache and betrayal did not disappear just because he was physically with me again, and increased exponentially with the amount of alcohol I drank. I decided I should try to attempt to drink twenty-one alcoholic beverages to kick off my twenty-first year. It was an impossible feat, of course, but I did my damnedest to reach that limit with Jason, and we became ruinously destructive later that night. We screamed, we cried, we fucked. He ended up sleeping between the sheets of my bed, while I stayed on top of the covers, shivering in the fetal position.

Hearing my story might actually have lightened Mike's load a bit.

Sometimes a moment of honest commiseration can make a burden slightly more bearable or at least less isolating.

But Mike and I weren't following our old routine. In that moment, I couldn't have recalled most of the details of my twenty-first birthday, not quickly enough to connect the two events when it was most relevant to him. It is possible that he and Amber might have had the fight even if he and I had connected over our matching romantic despair. But he was probably doubly injured when we didn't because he and his girlfriend were becoming distant at the exact same time he and his sister were drifting apart too.

The household was on only partially diplomatic terms the morning after my brother's fight with Amber. Mike's plan had been to come for his birthday and stay over Thanksgiving, and he hadn't given any indication that this had changed. He had not asked for his keys back. However, he seemed to be avoiding our parents, and I think they were avoiding him, too. My solution was simple: food. The doctors had agreed that I could drive within a five-mile radius—to the grocery store, to yoga classes—as long as there were no freeways involved. I hopped in the car and drove to a local fast-food joint called Everest to pick up the house special they referred to as "game time": french fries with chili, cheese, and pastrami on top. I had always thought it was revolting, but Mike's eyes lit up when I brought it home. It was his favorite. Although he clearly didn't want to talk about the night before with me, this hangover special loosened him up a bit.

He admitted he drank a lot more when Amber was around, and he told me that he had never drunk that much in his life. Since he had eventually blacked out, he wasn't even exactly sure what he did and said.

Might have proclaimed myself Princess Leia Organa of Alderaan, for all I know, Mike said weakly. He didn't deliver his joke with much oomph, but I could see he was trying to make me smile.

I was glad my brother had understood my peace offering. The french fries had also meant *I'm on your side. I can be on everyone's side.*

9

Justine lightly tapped the eraser side of her pencil on her desk a couple of times until she got my attention again.

Is something going on? she asked.

Sorry. Family stuff, I said. It's getting better, I think. I'm working on it.

It's really common, you know. Stress creates more word blockages for people with aphasia. By the way, how's the John Grisham book going?

Done, I said. Finally. But it took almost three months to finish it. You know, I realize that I am the one with the brain damage so I might be a poor judge here, but I also think that guy is a pretty lousy writer.

I gave Justine an exaggerated eye roll and she laughed.

Your gestures are very expressive, she said.

Lucky me, I said.

I'm not kidding, Lauren. You might not realize it, but you've got impressive tactics at your disposal when words fail you. Language influences, and is influenced by, gesture. Did you learn sign language at some point?

I was surprised by her question. I had always been animated, gesturing frequently with my hands, but no one had ever asked about it.

No, I said. I guess I move like this because of my acting-school background. And growing up in a house with a lot of drama.

Justine took her water glass over to the plants situated between the sliding doors.

I can recommend some American Sign Language classes, if you're ever interested, she said. What are you reading these days, now that Grisham has been crossed off the list?

Middlesex.

By Jeffrey Eugenides? she asked. That's certainly ambitious! She left her overturned water glass to drain its final drops into the fern.

Don't get too excited. I didn't say I understand it. My folks had it in their library so I just picked it up. All I can tell you about it is that the author used the word *quay* three times in a five-page span, and that seemed pretty unusual. Also, there is a character called Chapter Eleven, and in the eleventh chapter of the book I guess there is something that will be revealed about him. But maybe I'm missing something. Chapter Eleven. Is this book supposed to be self rential?

Self-referential? Justine clarified.

That's what I meant, I said. Self Ref-er-en-shul.

Your pronunciation of polysyllabic words is sounding better, she said. I can't help you with *Middlesex*, unfortunately, because I've never read it. But maybe I'll give you some short story reading assignments. The length will make it easier for you to follow the action. We can both read them, so we can have the same points of reference to discuss during our sessions.

Justine began to make notes about which stories she'd assign in coming weeks: H. G. Wells, Truman Capote, Thomas Wolfe, Guy de Maupassant, Sherwood Anderson, Edgar Allan Poe, and a few others.

Do you like F. Scott Fitzgerald? she asked me.

I think I used to love him, I replied. And his wife . . .

Zelda? Justine asked.

Yeah, I said. I liked her, too. I think I was in a play about her once.

A scholar and an actress all rolled into one, Justine said. When we go through the Fitzgerald story, I suspect you'll teach me more than I'll be teaching you.

It wasn't true. But I got caught up in her enthusiasm. Justine's willingness to engage with me in new ways and her intuition about how I might best respond had turned around a session that had started out somewhat raw.

10

It was two days before Thanksgiving when I got a phone call from BJ. His voice boomed through the receiver.

Did you get the good news? The register in BJ's voice started to slide up several octaves, until he was almost squealing. Materson is coming to America!

My parents, still grateful for the generosity they'd been shown in Edinburgh by the Patersons, had made it clear that Materson—or anyone else in their family—was welcome to visit us anytime. Materson was in his gap year between high school in Scotland and university in England. He was traveling the globe, with stops in New York, New Mexico, and California.

I didn't want to talk to BJ yet about what had just happened with my brother, but the discussion about Materson reminded me of Mike. Since the rupture and my return to the States, Materson and I had remained close. We communicated mostly through e-mail, but even as my language improved, I needed my dad to proofread all my correspondence. He would add all the words I had missed, and replace the words I had confused. With that constant mediation, it was impossible to be in close personal contact with anyone.

I told BJ I had received Materson's e-mail. The plan was to visit BJ and Laura in New York first, then he'd come out to LA to stay with us.

BJ couldn't wait to show him around.

It's hard to believe that that sweet boy is actually still a teenager, BJ said. When I was eighteen, I considered it my official duty to disappoint the nation-state of Texas by dyeing my hair and making out with boys. Laura was sneaking out to KISS concerts in catsuits and peeing in holy water. But our little Materson? His version of a teenage rebellion? He makes strangers pies.

As a matter of fact, Materson had just e-mailed the recipe for the banoffee pie he had made for all of us in Scotland. My mom and I planned to make it for Thanksgiving.

We started the baking early the next day. She looked preoccupied as she stirred her batter, an inarticulate worry rippling across her face as she glanced at the clock on the oven. She had hoped that Mike might help with the preparations for the holiday by taking care of basic chores, but they were still barely speaking. It was now two in the afternoon, and he was still sleeping upstairs. She knew the sound of the radio often distracted me so we worked silently, and I listened to the way she stirred and sighed.

In Scotland, Materson had used digestive biscuits to create the crust, but since they were hard to find in America, I was kneading graham crackers into the pie tin instead. The ribbons of toffee in my mother's saucepan were becoming a creamy brown. As soon as the candy thermometer hit 338 degrees Fahrenheit, she lifted the pan from the flame to bring the mixture over to me, but one of her red clogs got caught under the carpet runner at the counter. Her trip was slight, but in the split second before she regained her balance, the syrup started to drip toward the floor, and she reached out her hand for it.

For a moment, the caramel looked like a delicate brown bird, nesting in my mother's outstretched palm. But then her screams began. They were multiphonic and guttural, making the glass cabinets in the room rattle. As my mother thrust her hand into the cold tap water, I watched a layer of her skin slip away under the water as if she were taking off a glove. The burnt sugar could not be washed away, though. It was as sticky as it was molten.

She needed immediate help, but my response time was paralyzingly slow. I had always been her resourceful child, the one who could take charge, the one reliable in an emergency. But now, as much as I wanted to aid my mother, I was more transfixed by her metamorphosing hand than anything else.

I NEED HELP GODDAMMIT! she shrieked.

Realizing I would be no help, she bounded up the stairs. She bellowed the word *hospital*, and immediately I heard the thump of my brother leaping from his bed and the clang of his belt buckling. I broke from my spell and slowly put some ice into a dishtowel. When I handed it to my mom, she flung it into a bucket, which my brother filled with cold water. Her howls hadn't stopped. They'd gotten louder. She and my brother were out of the house in fewer than three minutes. I had to call my dad to tell him they were on their way to the hospital, but even that took a long time. I had to find the number written down somewhere. This was not the sort of thing I could remember anymore, especially under duress.

My dad and I arrived in different cars, and when we got to the hospital, my mother had been moved from the waiting area to a private room where the doctor was asking about the level of pain on a scale of one to ten. Her joints were white-locked, and her eyes were clenched shut. She bellowed: Ten! Ten!

Mike stayed next to her, rubbing her undamaged arm. He continued his reassuring touch through her second dose of morphine.

You are doing great, Mom, Mike said.

When the doctor came back in after a third dose, he again asked about her pain level.

She looked at him blearily, unable to focus her eyes this time: Ten? she asked him. Ten?

My brother adopted a soothing tone. I know it hurts, Momma, he whispered. But maybe it's a little better now, yeah? Maybe an eight?

Eight? Yeah, she slurred. Eights.

My dad kissed the top of my brother's head. Thank you, Mikey. You really saved the day.

I was grateful to see my family interacting again, huddled together close.

Later that night, I told Jonah about the hospital visit, praising Mike because he could get anywhere three times faster than I could, even if we took the same route. My mom had a quick decision to make and I was relieved she had chosen him. If it had been me driving . . . I said to Jonah. If we had gotten there any later, she would have needed a skin graft.

Does that mean you are able to drive again? Jonah asked.

Well, yeah, I said. But I thought Jonah was focusing on the wrong part of the story.

Isn't that great, though? My mom is doing well now and everyone in my family is talking again.

Yeah, I guess, Jonah said. But clearly your mom should've spoken to your brother earlier. If she had, she probably wouldn't have burned her hand.

The comment made me bristle. Whether or not this was true, this wasn't a well-packaged message from Jonah. It was the opposite of comforting. I had watched my mother suffer the worst pain of her life, her voice had unraveled into its shrillest octaves, and my brother had borne it all in a way I couldn't have. So, yes, my brother and mother could have had a heart-to-heart earlier, but Jonah was being too damn rational about all of this. New things were presenting themselves as part of my recovery, and though I still had to focus mainly on my rehabilitation, I wanted to tend to other obligations too. Didn't Jonah realize that I also had a family to look out for? Something about our emotional realities seemed radically misaligned then, and I was not sure how this had worked between us before. Would I need him to change? Did I need to?

11

A few days after the holiday hospital visit, Laura called to check up on me and see how my mother's hand was doing.

She won't be able to use it for a couple of weeks, I said. But it's not a permanent disability or anything.

I'm glad you brought up disability, actually, Laura said. Because I wanted to talk to you about getting disability payments from the state of New York. As opposed to your unemployment payments . . .

What do you mean? I asked her. What unemployment payments?

You were between jobs when you went to Europe, she said. Remember? You had worked at a hedge fund that closed right before you left, and your grad school had offered you a paid teaching position at Baruch College in the fall. But since there were a few months between those two paying gigs, you were receiving unemployment checks from New York State.`

That did ring a bell. And Laura went on to tell me I had received a few unemployment checks since the rupture.

But how? I asked. I didn't register online or anything.

Technically . . . you have, Laura said. When you were in the hospital, we all still thought you might be going back to work soon. And I kept thinking about how expensive your medical care was going to be. I'd seen you use the unemployment website before, and knew they sent direct deposits to your bank account. I guessed that your password would be the same as your e-mail. It was, so I filled in a few weeks of unemployment forms for you.

I hadn't thought about a bank statement in months. It hadn't even occurred to me, since my parents were covering everything financially.

I stopped filling in the forms when it was clear to everybody you couldn't go back to work right away, Laura continued. But I think you should contact the unemployment office now. Obviously, you should still be getting monthly subsidies, maybe even more money, but you should probably switch the unemployment payments to disability payments. Could be related departments, so might be an easy change.

That's a good idea, I said. Thank you for thinking of me. I'll get on that.

When I called the unemployment office of New York a few days later, I was transferred to a human voice surprisingly quickly, which was helpful since it was difficult for me to follow automated prompts. It seemed an auspicious beginning.

I told the woman who picked up the phone that I wanted to stop my unemployment payments as soon as possible.

Have you found a permanent position of employment, Miss Marks?

No, I said. But I had an accident. That's why I can't go to work now.

Uh-huh, the operator said, and I could hear her keyboard slowly tapping away. And what was the date of that injury? she asked.

I checked the paper next to me. I had written this information down before the phone call so I could read this script aloud. I was doing everything right.

August 23, 2007, I said.

There was a long pause from the woman, and then I heard her begin to type furiously.

Well, my records indicate that you have received payments since then. . . .

For some reason, I hadn't anticipated this response.

Oh. Yeah. But that's why I'm stopping now. Because I need help. Disability help.

The operator's voice became sharp: We're not talking about now, we are talking about then. And then, you received payments that you were not entitled to. Which means, Miss Marks, you have defrauded the state of New York.

It took a moment to recall if *defraud* was the opposite of *fraud*, or if they were synonymous. When I figured it out, I was horrified. If I had the intention of defrauding anyone, why would I expose myself? But I couldn't say that to this woman. I couldn't say anything, actually. My fragile language shattered under her attack, and even though I wanted to explain myself, words were failing me. The sounds I was making were a sludge of language. I probably said something like: *That if I don't can and I was I don't if that. Can't help, please I was if can't of If mean Help. Flumpppph Ssh You? Mom. No. Not? Uh. Uh. No. You? You?*

The woman over the phone was undeterred. If anything, she sounded more confident the more I floundered. Maybe she had never spoken to someone with aphasia before. Maybe she thought I was lying about this claim. But either way, she seemed to relish in the fact that I couldn't defend myself.

This is not the office of disability, Miss Marks, as you well know, she said. An accident or injury is purely irrelevant here. This is the unemployment office for the state of New York. If you are accepting unemployment payments, it is your responsibility to be ready and able to work at any moment, and you've already admitted that you were not at all ready or able to be employed at that time.

I just submitted to her insinuations, issued at a cruel speed, because I couldn't think of anything else I could do.

A month later, a bill arrived that I had to hand over to my mother sheepishly. Making that phone call had been a $1,342 mistake. My mom's forehead knit into a pattern of defeat.

You didn't do anything wrong, honey, she said. I'm not saying you did, and I know you want to do as much as you can for yourself. But you really have to let me handle this sort of thing in the future.

Neuropsychological evaluations can give a clearer picture of the challenges people face after a brain injury, and my mother was told this kind of examination was helpful for insurance purposes and filing disability claims. Since my ill-fated phone call to the unemployment office, placing me on federal disability had become a priority. My mother hurried to schedule another appointment at the University of Southern California Keck Medical Center in early December.

The neuropsychologist we met with was named Dr. Carol McCleary. She was a blonde woman with a Nordic build, and she arrived at our appointment dressed in an oversize cable-knit Christmas sweater and clunky holiday jewelry. She warned me that the test would take several hours.

I asked if I might be able to take the materials home when the testing concluded, so I could spend time on the areas where I struggled.

The sleigh-bells hanging from her ears jangled as she cocked her head. I'm afraid you can't take anything from the room since the test material is all copyrighted, she said. And it's not the kind of test you can study for, anyway. Even after the data has been acquired, the findings still need to be interpreted by our team. But you don't need to worry about any of that because I will be writing a detailed report about you.

This idea of having to be "interpreted" irked me, excluding my own sense of agency, especially since the ways in which I was going to be analyzed were not being disclosed to me.

But much like the language test with my speech therapist a couple of months earlier, the test itself was fascinating. The questions asked were both indirect and detailed, often based in procedures. For one task, I was asked to put pins in a board with my dominant hand and then with my less-dominant one. For other tasks, I had to arrange blocks, sequence letters and numbers, and remember a series backward and forward. I had to look at an angular drawing, which vaguely resembled a toy rocket resting on its side. I was only shown this piece of paper for a minute or two, then it was taken away, and I was asked to reproduce as much of the drawing as I could. This was the exact sort of thing I wanted to review when the test was over. What had I left out? And what did those exclusions mean? But I was never given an opportunity to compare the two figures side by side. McCleary had made it very clear that wasn't possible, so I just waited for the report to arrive in the mail.

When I received the paperwork a bit later, I saw that McCleary noted that my "general intellectual abilities" were in the "high average range," but I had issues with "multitasking" and "attention-shifting." She also wrote that the "neuropsychological protocol highlighted difficulties consistent with functions typically attributed to the frontal brain systems. Executive functioning was Ms. Marks's greatest area of weakness."

Executive functions are often closely linked with what is called *working memory*. Working memory is the ability to hold several items in mind for a short period of time, like learning a new person's name, or getting directions by the roadside. Often people remember these things by simply repeating them, encoding the new information in language, and then rehearsing it internally. On the test, I couldn't remember individual words in lists, but my recollections dramatically improved when those details were included inside an overall story, allowing me to visualize certain elements.

I learned that the frontal lobes are involved in processing judgments, calculating social norms, and inhibiting or expressing emotions, and are one of the many places where long-term memories are stored. They help govern things that make one person unique from another. When lobotomies were still common surgical practices—an ice pick inserted underneath the eyelid and into the frontal lobe—they effectively sliced away personalities, like a wiper blade on a windshield.

It disturbed me that McCleary had identified executive functioning as my area of weakness. If my executive functions made me *me*—who could I be without them?

However, I did like that McCleary mentioned that I had a "superior knowledge base, appreciation of abstract concepts, and knowledge of word meanings." I was pretty sure I knew what she was referring to: it had been one of my proudest moments during the testing. A research assistant had been going through a list of words aloud, asking me about their meanings. But she paused halfway down.

Hmm, she said. That's funny.

What's funny? I asked her.

Just a typo, I guess, she said. The word *hamlet* isn't capitalized here. . . .

That's because it doesn't have to be a person, I said, with a certainty that surprised me.

Oh really? she asked. What else could it be?

Hamlet. I hadn't thought of the word in ages. Jonah had played the role of Hamlet back in school, but I was positive there was another meaning as well. In my mind's eye, I slowly called up a scene of small houses with thatched roofs in a marshy medieval countryside.

A hamlet can also be . . . a location, I told her. Like a . . . village, or something.

I felt a surge of triumph. I was the girl with aphasia, correcting the language knowledge of the person administering my test. Later, though, I wondered if this had actually been orchestrated. It was a neuropsychological exam, and in an environment so tightly controlled, deception could be a legitimate tool in gathering certain information. But even if that was the case, I was pleased I passed this part of the test without fumbling.

Farther down on this report, I discovered a section that had nothing to do with this testing at all: Relevant History.

McCleary had written: "Ms. Marks was a doctoral student in theater before the hemorrhage." And for some reason, she had then added: "She describes herself as a writer."

I didn't remember telling McCleary I was a writer, but then, how else was I to describe myself? I had become a woman without a profession. I couldn't be an actor if I couldn't memorize. Couldn't be a PhD student if I couldn't read a textbook. But writing? That was one of the very few things I was still doing every day.

12

The winter holidays were fast approaching, and Jonah told me he was on a mission to make the best use of the time.

I'll be up at my dad's place in Seattle for a couple of weeks, he said. And as long as I am on the West Coast, I was just thinking how much I would love it if you would come join me up there.

The invitation caught me off guard. That might be nice, I said, seriously considering it. But I don't want to miss Christmas with my family.

You don't have to, he said. Have Christmas down in California, and celebrate New Year's in Washington with me.

It seemed like a shocking shift of reality. I hadn't left my parents' side since my stroke, but it had been a couple of months now, and maybe a trip would do me good. Yet, it seemed almost impossible to walk out the door of the home I was raised in and through the door of the home that Jonah had been raised in, within the span of just a few hours. Like a time traveler. If I was going to venture out this way, I felt I needed time to reflect on where I was coming from, and prepare myself for where I was going. I would need to ease into this type of trip.

There had been slight allowances for my driving recently, but there was no way I could get dispensation to go this far. Can I take a train up to Seattle? I asked Jonah.

Well, he hedged. I think so. If I remember right, the Coast Starlight comes all the way up from LA. But that's the super scenic route, Lauren. That would take you a couple of days. . . .

That sounds perfect, I said, happy that I could find a route that would give me plenty of time to think.

Just so you know, I can't stay in Washington for too long. If you decide to take the train, you'll probably cut into the time we could be spending together, Jonah replied, sounding a little disappointed. Are you sure you want to do it that way?

That was, I suspect, a hint. Jonah was asking me to reconsider my travel plans, so we could capitalize on all his time away from the East Coast. He already had a distinct kind of trip in mind, but I was trying to conceive of my own. For me to be fully sympathetic to his desires, I'd have to consider our positions side by side. I would have to imagine multiple scenarios, playing them out to their hypothetical conclusions. My Theory of Mind wasn't sophisticated enough for that, or as my neuropsychologist had mentioned, I just wasn't good at multitasking. If I was going to make a decision about a path forward, I only had room for my own reality.

I'd like to see you, I said. But I think I have to do my travel slowly.

As long as you're coming, I'll take what I can get, he said, sounding pleased. And he turned a corner in our conversation, employing an entirely different register of his voice. You know, he said. If I have to wait even longer to see you . . . maybe you could give a guy a break. You could tide him over with a picture or two.

I wasn't totally sure what his tonal shift indicated, or what he was suggesting exactly. Pictures? I asked him to repeat himself.

Oh come on, Lo, he said. You know what I mean. It's been a long time since I've seen you. Been near you . . .

Sure, I said. I guess I could find some photo of me in my mom's albums. . . .

Jonah laughed. Whoa. I certainly hope you wouldn't find the kind of picture *I'd* like in your mom's collections.

Oh no? I asked. Why's that?

Ahem. Well. Okay. Jonah laughed again, but this time a little nervously. Didn't realize I had to be so explicit here. I was just suggesting that you could take a picture of yourself. And I just wouldn't especially complain, if this photo turned out to be a little . . . racy.

I immediately thought of the Santa Anita Racetrack, which had been across the street from my elementary school. We used to do our gym laps in their parking lot. Then I remembered there was another meaning to the word *racy*.

As I started to work through the facets of the meaning internally, Jonah noted my silence and started to backpedal. Of course, if you don't want to take the picture, please don't do that, he said. It's really not important.

I told him that I might have to think about it.

No problem. Only if the spirit moves you, he said. I heard the sound of the refrigerator door opening and the clunk of a plastic pitcher, pouring a glass of water.

You're gonna love it up in Seattle, Lauren. It's so clean. And green everywhere. Unlike New York, it was built at a human scale. Just beautiful. Like my beautiful girl.

Before I fell asleep that night, I brought my camera to my bedside and attempted to take a few pictures of myself. I was nude except for my black hip-huggers. There was nothing explicit, only white curves against red sheets. But my gaze looked so confused in every shot. It wasn't at all alluring or inviting, or if it was, I was a poor judge of it. Instead, my eyes kept looking up as if they were asking a question. In earlier stages of my relationship with Jonah, a provocative prompt from him was an opening move into a mutual flirtation, which would then escalate into a chemical crave. This time, though, I didn't feel any of that urgency. And even though I didn't want Jonah to be disappointed, I decided against sending the pictures. I kept trying to imagine being with him, to visualize our reunion in his father's house.

But I simply couldn't. I got hung up on details. How big was the living room? Does the lawn have a porch? I had no template to build on. In the years Jonah and I had dated in New York, I had never been to Washington. He had never asked me to join him. Now he seemed more excited about this trip than I was. I was sure there was a possibility that I could *become* excited, when the time came. The old sensations, whatever they might have been, could rekindle. Maybe soon. Maybe in Seattle. But, in the meantime, I used my journal to write my way to the other side of my unease.

Jonah and I had seen each other right before I left for Paris. We both had plans to leave the city that summer: me for the European tour, him for Alaska.

We ate at our favorite bistro in the West Village, Tartine, which had a bring-your-own-booze policy. We quickly drank a very big and very cheap bottle of red wine, and ended up on the far side of tipsy. It had been an intimate night out, but as we arrived at the Union Square subway, Jonah told me he wanted to sleep at his place that night, and I took that to mean that I wasn't invited. Being alone didn't normally upset me, but we wouldn't be seeing each other for two and a half months. Why didn't he want to spend our last few nights together? In protest, I crossed my arms and planted myself on a bench. A light rain had already started to fall, and though my teeth began to chatter, I was unwilling to get up. Jonah remained standing.

I wanted him to change his mind, but more than that, I wanted an explanation. Any explanation. An alcohol-fueled insecurity was bringing out a neurotic streak in me, my ability to be agonizingly self-critical. And when I felt I might be failing at something, my frantic mind could quickly veer toward panic or despair, and my inner voice would go into overdrive. *Why was he being so withholding? Was he leaving me that night so he could see another woman?*

Any reassurance from Jonah could have stopped me from going down this rabbit hole, but he just stood there.

I want to go home. He shrugged. So I am going home.

Though we were prone to debates and disagreements, Jonah and I rarely fought, at least not in the traditional sense—unlike most couples, we didn't snap at each other and never shouted. We shared a strong sense of curiosity and loved asking questions about the world, but we used different manners of inquiry when answering these questions, and we often arrived at very different conclusions. I loved that Jonah spoke his mind regardless of popular view. After all, it was what had drawn me to him in the first place. It was wonderful when we fought the good fight on the same side, and what others perceived as his obstinacy, I saw as conviction. But his particular brand of insistence was so uncompromising it could be alienating to others. Friends had dropped out of his life, and there were even a few directors who didn't work with him anymore because of it. He would defend his positions on matters of capital T truth, and if people were wounded as a byproduct of his scrutiny, he paid very little attention to that. But he could never be as objective as he wanted to be. He suffered from unpredictable mood swings, and these tempers kept him tethered to the limits of his very subjective experience, something all people are prey to. However challenging these traits might have been, there were plenty of reasons I was drawn to the extremity of his personality. In the beginning of our relationship, I was a somewhat temperamental force myself. Cocky, even. However, being Jonah's partner while he experienced these swings had made me much more empathetic to him. Unfortunately, in the moments in which he'd become most detached, I'd want to draw closer.

As I sat at the station in Union Square, I blinked raindrops off my eyelashes, trying to stifle a quiver in my voice.

Why does it have to be so difficult between us? I asked him. All of this. We love each other, but at this point in our relationship, shouldn't we be better partners?

Partners, huh, he said. An odd term to use. Like your parents? His tone was lacking any sympathy, drained of its intonation as well. It would frustrate me to no end when he sounded like that. Privately, I referred to this as his "robot voice."

While the wine had made me sappy, it had made him stoic. Well, we're not setting up an advertising agency together, if that's what you mean, Jonah said. So is that what you are really talking about?

At the mention of my parents, I became convinced that Jonah was suggesting that this was my slant way of broaching the topic of marriage. I was almost twenty-seven. I didn't know if I wanted to marry Jonah, didn't know if I wanted to marry anyone. But, in my petulant boozy stupor, I became utterly convinced that *he* should want to marry *me*. And at that hour of the night, I didn't want to be analyzed or reasoned with. I wanted to be small as a dime, so Jonah could slip me into his coat pocket and carry me home.

Instead, I descended into the subway station alone, and wrung out my dripping skirt, thinking that this might be the beginning of an end for us. It wouldn't have been our first separation, but it had the potential to be the final one.

Jonah called me the next day, though. He was in a much better mood, kinder, and we both apologized for our behavior. He even brought over a present wrapped for my birthday, an occasion that would take place while we were thousands of miles away from each other. And we made up in our usual way—in bed.

13

In mid-December, I had another consult with Dr. Russin, in her office on a leafy Pasadena street. She had asked me to come by so we could talk about a somewhat sensitive subject.

There's no specific cause for concern, she said as we sat down. But during the treatment of your ruptured aneurysm, the CT scan in Edinburgh detected something of note. You seem to have another aneurysm as well.

The news came as a shock. I stared at her in teary disbelief, hoping I had misunderstood.

I have *two* aneurysms in my brain?

It appears so, but the second is quite small, she said, looking at her clipboard. You need to remember lots of people have aneurysms. Not all of them rupture. In fact, most don't. And this one is much smaller than the first. We just have to keep an eye on it.

That wasn't much of a consolation. After all the doctor's visits, I'd learned that location was everything inside the skull. My first aneurysm had been near the language centers of the brain, and as a result, the damage had dramatically reshaped my ability to use language and affected my entire world. If there was another rupture in a different part of my brain, what

else could be compromised? My motor skills? My eyesight? My capacity
to reason morally?

Suddenly, I thought of Ralph Waldo Emerson, the father of American
Transcendentalism; I had recently discovered that in his later years, he too
had had aphasia. It was a progressive form that appeared to have developed
alongside his Alzheimer's, though at the time that disease did not yet have
a name. In *On Nature*, he had written:

> "Standing on the bare ground,—my head bathed by the blithe air, and
> uplifted into infinite space,—all mean egotism vanishes. I become
> a transparent eye-ball; I am nothing; I see all; the currents of the
> Universal Being circulate through me; I am part or particle of God."

It gave me comfort that near the end of Emerson's life, he somewhat
became that figure he'd once written about, less like a man, more like a
gaze. He couldn't write in his later years or read without assistance. When
he picked up one of his own books, he couldn't even identify the author.
There was no medical recourse for treating his condition, though it was
reported that as his intellectual, cognitive, and executive functions degen-
erated, his humor never soured. Long after the onset of his dementia, an
acquaintance asked how he was feeling. He responded by saying, "Quite
well. I have lost my mental faculties, but am perfectly well."

If there was to be another change in the topography of my brain, I
prayed my cortical map would be changed for the better. *Let me be Emerso-
nion*, I thought. *Let me become grateful, even for my lack.*

> *what if i begin again. find my losses grea the same or greater than this
> time? let me be like emerson; thankful for his* dimension *(?). when he
> orients for a moment, long enough to answer the question "how are doing"
> and to reply "i have lost my mental faculties, but I'm perfectly well, thank
> you."*

14

I was jumping up and down on my mother's plush white couch—in my arms was a story Justine had photocopied for me. Though I had read the pages back in high school, everything about it on this go-around was breathtakingly new. "A Soldier's Home" was changing everything. I scurried to the phone to call Grace.

Grace, I can read this! I exclaimed. I mean, I can actually *read* this!

She laughed. Grace had been patient with my outbursts over the last few months, and she encouraged me to contact her when I encountered any new developments in my language.

This sounds great, she said, but maybe you can catch me up first.

I explained that I was reading Hemingway for speech therapy. A story from *In Our Time*.

There is this scene with Krebs in his parents' home after the war, I explained to her. His mother is telling him not to muss his father's paper, but he could probably borrow his car. Like he is still a kid. After what Krebs has just gone through, this scene—it's all ludicrous, right?

Definitely, Grace said. And purposely so.

But what is so amazing is that Hemingway doesn't say anything about the scope of the change that's taken place, I continued. And Krebs doesn't say anything about that either. There is a whole atmosphere apart from the words on the page.

Yeah, Hemingway is famous for his sparse language, Grace said approvingly. Leaving things to the reader's imagination.

It's perfect, I said. Even the name of the story is perfect, isn't it? "A Soldier's Home"? Because that's not even possible, right? There is no such thing as *home* for a soldier. Not anymore. I was nearly breathless.

Grace, I said. There is this thing that is not *on* the page here, but what *could have been* on the page. You know? I don't know what to call it exactly. But it's the entire story not being told. . . .

Are you talking about reading between the lines? Grace asked. Like subtext?

Subtext—that's it! I started jumping again. That is *exactly* it! *Sub*-text. This revelation fully winded me.

I hadn't had this skill since the aneurysm's rupture. Until this very second, I *couldn't* read between the lines. And the craziest thing is I didn't know I had lost that ability.

That's . . . Wow. I don't know, Grace said. That's pretty hard for me to imagine, so this must be really disorienting for you.

I don't know what it is. I paused. It's amazing, actually. But now that I have this skill back, it feels dangerous too. Because now I have something too precious to lose.

Wish I could be a fly on the wall during your speech therapy! Grace said. I might even be able to pick up some tips for my own sessions at the writing center.

Grace had all but finished the course requirements for her PhD in English at Columbia University, and she was working as the assistant director in the writing center on campus.

It's just interesting to see the building blocks of language from this vantage point, she continued. Surprising to think about the sort of things you are working on.

Mainly I've been working on this essay, I said. Hours every day. And still it's taking months to finish.

Hmm. You've mentioned it before, she said. I'd love to see it sometime.

You would? I asked, a little surprised.

Of course, silly. It would be much more fun than putting together the annual report for the writing center, that's for sure.

Grace told me that she was headed back to California for the holidays.

Why don't you send a draft of your essay before I get there? she suggested. Then we can discuss it in person.

The night before Christmas Eve, we met at Grace's parents' condo in Arcadia and headed down to the basement office to chat. For years, the two of us had exchanged our work, providing feedback and volleying back and forth to clarify our ideas. We grabbed mismatched chairs and faced each other like chess pieces. She took out my essay, but for some reason, she seemed nervous.

I'm not sure how to begin, she said. And I noticed her tone sounded uncertain, too.

Just tell me what you think, I said.

Well . . . It's kind of . . . It's sort of . . . She took a moment to compose herself. I'm just going to talk to you like someone who has just come through the doors of the writing center, is that okay? In third person. I think it's important to deal with text impersonally sometimes. That's what you want, right?

Sure! I said eagerly. Go ahead.

This essay has many impressive attributes, she began, which are in no small part offering a glimpse into an experience most people will never have. But I have some concerns, I guess. Because the piece strikes me as . . . incomplete.

Dutifully, I started to take notes. Is my grammar so bad? I asked.

No, no. It's something else, she said. She flipped to a page she highlighted, and then read something I had written back to me:

I started hearing from dozens of people, some I hadn't heard from
in years. The tenor of all the emails, that my parents read me aloud from
the inclined bed, was approximately the same, eerily similar, "Get well
soon," "You'll be back to your old self again in no time," and, always,
"Persevere!"

Over these two months since the aneurysm I have started to a
incubate an uneasiness with these cheers of "perseverance." And I've
started to believe that it might be advising me badly. I take even the
issue with the timbre used of the well-wishers. Disappoint. Condolences.
Regret. Unexpectedly, I struggle with these correspondences. I couldn't
possibly describe this experience I've had, and I'm still having. And all
of its sub-sets of experiences. I might begin with: Altering. Exhilarating.
Ineffable.

Grace stopped there. Now see, there is this big meta-story missing for
me, she explained. The author of this piece is being supported entirely by
a network of people around her, yet she doesn't discuss this web of support at all. Her statements strike me as insensitive or, at least, incredibly
unaware.

I was a little confused. Well, those people aren't really the point of the
piece for m . . . I mean, the author, I said a bit defensively. She is incredibly
grateful for everyone, of course. But the essay is about the complications of
perseverance, and about words themselves. I pointed out another section in
the essay to prove my point, and read it to Grace.

No one has asked about this, so I can only believe that they don't
know to question it, about the gift of wordlessness. The silence, the
stillness, the absence of words, is a once in a lifetime experience. In
Edinburgh I found quietness I had never believed existed. A nothing
mind, a fragment of flotsam. Often, I don't conjure a full thought for
hours at a time, and would have the words to keep or shape it when it
came. I am a buoyant child's bath toy, bobbing along unconcerned atop of
an expanse of an unknown sea.

But Grace countered that. Even that excerpt deals with other people, she said. Look at the beginning of the paragraph: "No one has asked" the author something. That means that these expectations about perseverance appear to come from sources *outside* her. It echoes back to the group who "might be advising her badly." Other people are directly implicated in this piece, as kind of, maligning sources.

That's not the intent at all, I protested. It's just like Krebs, a soldier with no home to come home to.

But this author is not a soldier, Grace said. And this is not a war.

I took a moment. I understood she was being literal, but I felt Grace was missing something. Maybe my aphasia didn't involve guns or uniforms, but I had undergone a trauma that had caused an unexpected and profound change in my worldview. Like Krebs, this powerful experience had rendered me, in the eyes of others, fragile and in need of constant supervision and care.

Okay. Guess I see your point, I said. But even with all of this amazing personal support, what if the author feels like this is a small part of something much bigger? What if she feels her experience is somewhat fateful? As if the whole thing was . . . meant to be.

The fluorescent bulb above us flickered and Grace's blue-green eyes twitched. Well, since that idea doesn't jive with my worldview as a reader, the writer would become an unreliable narrator to me. She read again from the essay:

> *I bristle even writing the word "recovery." I have a thorny relationship with its semantics. Re-turn. Re-member. Re-cover. Every word implies getting back, but there is no back to go to. This is not a physical injury like a sprain or break, which needs to be mended. There is no pain and there is no cure, and this is as it should be. This is not a revival, but a genesis.*

Don't you see how problematic this is? Grace shook her head. Because text like that makes me think the author is sick and just wants to stay sick.

For almost a full minute after she said that, there was no sound in that basement in Arcadia, except the rolling buzz of the fluorescent tubes on the ceiling.

The Girl I Used to Be would have agonized over such a scathing interpretation of herself, especially from someone she so deeply admired. But in this new life, I was more curious than upset. My interactions with Justine about this essay had mainly consisted of agreement and encouragement. The way Grace had received this piece presented a wholly unexpected challenge. Although I already knew my language could be wobbly, it hadn't occurred to me that even after all that time on my own, selecting what I thought were the exact right words, my actual message could still be misunderstood.

Would you let me expand on my final point, actually? Grace asked, her tender eyes starting to fill. It's not my impression that the writer won't physically recover. She is well on the road already—it's apparent in her text. But this author has some unreasonable viewpoints, and some people might be concerned that she won't recover from those ways of thinking.

This was an incredible thing to consider. Grace had known so much about me for so long, and vice versa. We'd forged our own senses of self, side by side, and in no small part, our friendship was based around the language we used together. And I don't think we'd ever been more linguistically disconnected than we were in this moment. The essay had simultaneously done much more and much less than I thought it would. It was meant to be all about words, but Grace had added something to it that I had not even been aware of: this piece of writing put language first and people second.

Later that night, I continued to ask the questions of myself that Grace had asked of me. I wanted to understand what had actually happened between us. And what I wasn't able to say in my interaction with her in person became a lengthy exploration in my journal.

in this essay itself..in words, I am in returning to the (world of words)
~~each utterance~~ every sentence every phrase to me are ~~seem supreme~~

profoundly gratifying. with naked experience, my dressing it ~~tail~~ words
that tailor (fit) to it.

communities people perceive us
I tell my good friend that in some ways I am like—>a soldier returning
~~from the war~~ to the soldier's home. ~~the to~~ find ~~it that~~ the world he knew
~~doesn't have seem to fit~~ before, and expected it ~~be~~ to be . . .

She says gravely "But you weren't in a war"—>Perhaps she is right. Some
analogies are verbodden. Each sufferer to each singular condition.

15

Over Christmas, some of our extended family came in from Minnesota to celebrate the holiday with us. I expected that the influx of so many bodies and sounds would overwhelm me, but I did a little better than I had when my cousins had come from San Diego. I didn't seek out places to hide, at least. Everyone was their vacation self and instead of rushing about, people adopted a leisurely pace, wandering through the house in their pajamas. It was a tempo that matched my own inner speed nicely. Michael had come back down from Monterey, and though he told me he had patched things up with Amber, he was wise enough not to invite her over. We all spent a cozy night together playing board games by the fire, my grandmother and me sipping cider from the sidelines. The next day, I was on the train to see Jonah.

On the Coast Starlight, I spent the majority of my time in the observation car, its walls made entirely of glass, letting the landscape wash over me. I collapsed into the rocking click-clack of the carriages; the Quiet had become harder to access as my inner and outer voices had become louder, but I now was able to drift in and out of it with no effort at all.

With thirty-five hours to kill, I thought a lot about Paris.

• • •

For such an ancient city, the buildings in Paris were much cleaner than I had expected them to be, or at least they were in the part of town where Krass was subletting. The structures were as decorative and ornate as petit fours. I loved Krass's apartment, and staying there made me feel like less of a tourist and more like a traveler. I spent as much time as I could wandering around the city, taking it all in. Krass encouraged my solo expeditions, but I loved seeing the sights with him, too. Walking by his side, every block was enriched with a storied piece of history. His knowledge of the city was inspiring, and only added to its allure.

Krass was a pronounced aesthete and his philosophical musings usually drifted toward art, beauty, or sex. As a teacher, he often told his pupils to go to more museums and eat more delicious food, but he also advised them to fall in love more and have more sex. The way he spoke so freely shocked a few students, and in professor evaluations, some even remarked how "Krass" lived up to his name. But it was theater school, and rules of conduct and decorum were pretty lax. Krass rarely discussed the details of his own escapades, but he insisted that monogamy was overrated and should generally be avoided.

And, on principle, I espoused the same liberal ideology as Krass.

During the early stages of my relationship with Jonah, I told him that we shouldn't be exclusive. It was an odd condition to lay down in the beginning, especially since things were going well between us, and Jonah was still so smitten. He was crushed that I had even suggested it, probably assuming I thought of him as inadequate in some way, or that I wanted to be able to see several other men concurrently. That was not the case. At the time, I could count all of my sexual partners on one hand, and when I had committed to someone, I never once cheated on them. However, I strongly linked sexual autonomy to self-reliance. Monogamy was too much like ownership, especially for women. I didn't want any of my relationships to form such slavish attachments.

In general, I distrusted the desire for ready-made coupledom. It was ridiculous to me that two different people were expected to combine all their desires, hopes, and worldviews as soon as they paired up. I had always wanted my independence. I thought the terms *boyfriend* and *girlfriend* were too possessive, and employed the term *lover* much more often. It was a reciprocal word, an active word that described what we did, as opposed to what we were.

But, my rules of autonomy didn't last long. In the first few months with Jonah, I let myself feel worldly, and very much in control. At some point soon after that, though, I stopped playing the freewheeling character and let myself become much more attached. Jonah adored me, I adored him, and it turned out that I adored being adored. He wrote me love notes, which I treasured. It was a committed and monogamous relationship for a long time, and we never really discussed what the protocol would be if that dynamic changed.

It did change, of course. I don't know the hour or the day exactly, but about two years into our relationship, Jonah took the "advice" I had given him at the beginning of our relationship and slept with another woman. And it was not a one-night thing. Technically, he didn't lie about it. In fact, he was almost pathologically honest, but he did wait until I asked him about it. When I first found out, my heart turned so heavy it felt it might plummet straight through my body like a ten-ton anchor. We talked about the affair. I don't remember much about the conversation, but I seriously doubt I was able to keep a dispassionate veneer. He knew I was hurt, and I knew he never wanted that. Still, I felt I couldn't fully blame him. I'd introduced the possibility of this, and now I had to walk that walk. If I insisted on a monogamous relationship from this point on, I would have to reverse my former convictions. It felt like hypocrisy, like I was failing at feminism or something. I simply wasn't willing to do that. So I didn't even try to negotiate terms about the future of our relationship, which had plenty of ups and downs after that. Jonah and I broke up more than once, but we would also reunite for long and euphoric stretches too. Several months before I left for Paris, Jonah had become romantically involved with another woman—a friend of a friend—and this specific interaction was much more than a fleeting dalliance. Once again, I was confronted with the nettles of my supposed "empowered" rhetoric. Ostensibly, Jonah and I had the same amount of agency in pursuing the parameters of our close, but potentially non-monogamous, relationship. Jonah had slept with several women while we were still deeply involved, embarking on very short-lived affairs with all of them. But me? Since our pairing up as a couple, I had slept with one other man, on one night, and never again. I was somewhat disappointed to find out that my default was that of a monogamist.

Jonah and the newest woman stopped seeing each other months before I left the States, but this recent fracture of our intimacy still left its shards in me. I brought it up with Krass, but only in the broadest ways. He cared about my concerns, but he didn't understand why I would even *want* to commit myself to Jonah, or to anyone else, at my age. If I forced Krass to comment on my ongoing romantic tug-of-war, he would sigh, and remark on how disappointingly heteronormative it was.

It wasn't that Krass didn't believe in love, quite the opposite. He loved love, and perhaps it was just the love of art that bewitched him the most. This was evident the day he took me to Montparnasse. One of his favorite museums was there, nestled among still-functioning artists' galleries and lofts. Inside, he lingered over the informal photographs before planting himself in front of a picture of Kiki du Montparnasse, whom he called the patron saint of the neighborhood. He explained that she had modeled for dozens of pieces in this museum alone. She was the back in Man Ray's *Le Violon d'Ingres*, and it was her bronze bust that sat in the lobby. Krass had been reading a biography of the district, which also chronicled Kiki's love affairs. He pointed at a picture of Kiki wearing a wilted fox wrap, looking especially hungover.

You should take on her gig! Krass said, as if he were giving me an actual job recommendation. You've got the same angular bob. And the same red lipstick. To be a proper artist's muse, you'd have to take a lot of lovers, and swig a lot of martinis, but that's not too bad if you ask me.

Though I never took this suggestion seriously, I appreciated Krass's input, and it did make me think. I was in the city of Sartre and Beauvoir, for God's sake. Jonah and I hadn't exactly discussed the state of our relationship after the Union Square incident the month before, and if I was so dissatisfied with the way things were going, why couldn't I exploit some of the "flexibility" in our relationship model myself? I daydreamed about indulging the whims of my promiscuous Parisian alter ego, but my heart just wasn't in it. I had already discovered that I had an almost-destructive talent for devotion. It was just hard to pursue someone, or even be interested in someone, when another figure loomed so large in my imagination. In Europe, I didn't want to breach my relationship with Jonah, as long as we were still having one.

When my train pulled into the Seattle station, cold air rushed through the open carriage door. I slipped my winter coat on, and as I got off the train, Jonah was waiting for me just as he'd promised.

It was a short drive to his family home in Green Lake, but his father and sister were already in bed when we arrived. Jonah led me into the dark living room. The plastic tree was the size of a lawn gnome, sitting on a coffee table in the corner, its twinkling colored bulbs the only source of light.

I have something for you, Jonah whispered. And, from under the tree, he pulled out a long, blue velvet box.

Open it, he said.

Inside was a delicate chain with a silver pendant. It showed a pair of scissors on it, with an engraving that read, "We Part to Meet Again."

It's an analogy! I said, enthused by delight. I've been learning about those! You and I are like the blades of the scissors, right?

Thought you might enjoy that. Jonah beamed.

I feel silly now, I said, hugging him. I took a Christmas tin out of my duffle. I just made fudge for you and your family. I've got a present for you, too, but something small.

As Jonah unwrapped the paper, he found a used book about the James Bond movies.

Ah, he said, looking pleased. So you remember our Bond-a-thons, eh?

I nodded. We saw all the movies together, didn't we?

Well, *I* saw the movies. *You* mainly slept through them. But . . . His voice perked up. We can make up for lost time and continue our *Bonding* experience. Not tonight, of course. You've had a long journey and you must be tired.

I was exhausted, but I had no idea where to put my bag.

Come bring it into my bedroom, he said.

Is that where I am staying? I asked. With you?

Where else? Jonah laughed. Unless you have any objections?

No. It's not that, I said. We just hadn't really talked about sleeping arrangements. . . .

Sorry, I thought it was a given, he said. There isn't even a guest room in this house. I assumed the sleeping arrangements would be the same as it would be in New York, you in my bed, and me right next to you. Just like always. Is that okay?

Everything was okay and it wasn't. I had never been in this space before, I hardly knew his family, so I didn't know how to behave or interact with them yet, and I still didn't know how to interact or behave with Jonah, either. And his comment about "just like always" didn't minimize my discomfort. He had an effortless access to a long and detailed history of us that I simply did not have. But I was excited nonetheless.

Jonah took me down a passageway lined with potted plants to a bedroom with a single twin bed inside. A cat darted through the open door.

Well, here is the famous Neutron you've heard so much about, Jonah said, giving her a generous pet before shooing her away. But we don't need a chaperone tonight, Neutie. Three's a crowd.

The cat can stay, I said, a little relieved. Even though I was vaguely allergic, I at least knew how to behave around a cat.

I unzipped my jacket and Jonah slowly unbuttoned my sweater. I peeled off my black tights, and lay down with him. Strangely, I don't remember if Jonah and I got any more intimate that night. We certainly did on this trip, but what I remember most from the first evening was my insomnia.

Jonah fell asleep easily, with me in a tight grip. Though I had loved feeling his arms around me back in New York, his body heat was unbearable in that tight, slim Seattle bed. I unpeeled Jonah's knee from my thigh, his elbow from my torso, but his sleeping body kept seizing me in another bony entrapment. Occasionally, my nose would be hit by the swish of a cat's tail. Instead of sleeping, I watched the moonlight creep across the plaster ceiling until I heard Jonah's dad leave for work soon after dawn. That was when I crept downstairs.

Midmorning, Jonah found me in the breakfast nook, his face creased with pillow marks. I was picking my way through book one of Casanova's memoirs, *The History of My Life*, which I had brought for the train ride. Reading was still problematic, so I had to be selective with what I chose. I had been attempting some general articles about the brain and aphasia, but I didn't understand most of the scientific and medical terms yet. Although Casanova's language was old, his memoir was a sequential story, with vivid descriptions and straightforward storytelling. There was nothing that required any major interpretation on my part, which made reading easier for me. Jonah jokingly approved of the salacious subject matter I'd chosen.

It's not like that, I protested. Sex is only a very small part of the book.

I told Jonah how Casanova was born poor, and had lost and built his fortune several times over the course of his life. He was a soldier, spy, and cabalist. He pioneered one of the first national lotteries, in addition to being a confidant of popes. He was imprisoned in a few countries and broke out of more than one jail. In many ways, he made his entire career out of fantastic failures, and every time, he was forced to begin again. His new lives were often even more fraught with conflict than the ones before it. I loved how he was unapologetic about his upheavals. Somehow, I completely skipped over the people he hurt in the process, and the lives he was too careless with. But his fearless drive for change, and his constant adaptability, were the traits that impressed me most, serving as a reminder to me that a person could live several lifetimes in a single body. These often-ignored aspects of Casanova occupied my thoughts, and appeared in my writings as well. . . .

In my last life, I so strived to attain perfection. In this one, I embrace my flaws like a loved friend.

this period could warrants the canonization of casanova. if he had one
singular governing principle ~~there~~ that was ~~of wholeheartedly~~ his lack
of fear for failure. his experience illustrated that his ability to change. to
have his failures as great as his successes.

Seattle's low and heavy clouds made its tallest buildings look like shoulders without heads, and this skyline reflected my own peculiar brand of haze. After spending so much time by myself since the rupture, it was genuinely odd to me to be paired up again, with very little exertion on my part. I simply arrived in a location in the world and I had a ready-made boyfriend. When Jonah had visited me in Edinburgh, he had been my traveling companion and nothing more. Now we were lovers again. This dynamic was infused with exhilarating potential and flirtation. But, I couldn't quite lose the unsettling sense of imbalance—Jonah still felt very new to me, and that feeling was not mutual.

Jonah drove us everywhere in the city. The Elliot Bay Bookstore, Pier 54, the Space Needle. He pointed out his old schools and theaters. He took me whale watching, got us massages, found the highest hill to watch the New Year's fireworks display, and made sure I sampled the best clam chowder in town. I hadn't come to Seattle with any plans and I was impressed with him playing the role of guide, but I also would have been pleased with so much less. I got the sense that he had tailored these tourist activities to my tastes specifically, but I wasn't sure what my tastes had been before, or if they were the same now. And the only time Jonah appeared to be aware of shifts in my preferences was when we ordered at restaurants and cafés. He noticed changes in my food choices. I didn't like anything with too much salt, and craved apples and rare steaks. Jonah said he remembered me preferring vegetarian fare, with a special love for corn chips and guacamole. And though we drank a few cocktails in Seattle, he remarked that I never actually requested my favorite drinks, and I didn't drink nearly as much of anything.

Then there was my voice. I had gotten much better at hearing myself when I spoke, and was making fewer mistakes in my speech. But I was out of my comfort zone. I was used to hearing myself with my family, with a doctor, with a therapist. Now in different locales and surrounded by new people, there was an onslaught of stimuli, and I was required to employ a new vocabulary. Sometimes I had word-finding delays. But other times, language would come up more automatically, like a reflex. Then I would second-guess this burst of fluency. I also had such an ache to put myself in context. *Had I always sounded like this? Did I sound odd to anyone else?* Jonah found it endearing when I asked him questions about how my speech was being received by people around me, and by him specifically. He did his best to be accommodating, but this didn't stop the thousands of daily shocks to my system.

Jonah's family home was another environment that took a lot of getting used to. It was not a familiar dynamic. While my family was open and overly involved in one another's affairs, his was reserved and somewhat disconnected. Meals were rarely shared and there were a lot of closed doors. I hardly saw Jonah's sister, and spent only slightly more time with his dad. Everyone was respectful of me, and of one another's space, but to such an extent that it felt like they lived in their own personal apartments. Only occasionally would someone end up passing through a communal area. To me, it felt like no one was in charge and the absence of a mother's presence was palpable.

The morning of my departure, Jonah and I arrived on the train platform a few minutes early. It was windy, so Jonah pulled up the oversize collar of my heavy coat.

See what I did there? he asked. Your little genius engineered a makeshift kissing booth. Jonah brought his face close to mine, inside our new woolen enclosure. Our chapped, wintery lips ground like mortar and pestle. Rough becoming smooth.

I don't want to let you go, Jonah said. And I am only going to do so on the condition that the next time I see you, we can be together for a lot longer.

Jonah's statement surprised me. I hadn't regretted coming up to Seattle in the slightest, but I wouldn't have wanted to stay any longer. I felt that both of us were looking forward to spending some time alone. Apparently, Jonah didn't share the sentiment.

I didn't want to overstay my welcome, I told him.

You are killing me here, Lauren. You know I love you, I do. But you almost spent as many days on the train as you spent in Seattle.

The rails beside us buzzed, and a distant train became visible. Glad you came up for New Year's, though, Jonah said, and kissed my forehead. 2008 is starting out pretty good, I'd say.

Grace had called the people around me a web of support, and I could see now what she had meant. I had been beyond lucky that most of my loved ones had not distanced themselves from me after the stroke. But this came with a strange set of corollaries because people were seeing so many aspects of me that I didn't see in myself. They were assuming and expecting and applying my wants before I could even establish them myself. And they weren't seeing the parts of me that I felt were the most pronounced, the things I was actually able to identify. This was never as obvious as it was with Jonah. In Seattle, it had been impossible to keep up with these multiple versions of myself in real time, so I tried to keep up with Jonah's version of me instead. And I felt like I did a good job of it, eventually. He was putting so much effort into our romance, and although I found the attention a bit overwhelming, it honestly made me happy to see him happy.

I snuggled against Jonah's neck before I boarded the train. On the steps, I quickly turned around and attempted to say a final word, but had to speak over the din around us. I pointed at my necklace—and promised him: We part to meet again.

16

In my neurologist's exam room, Seattle felt like a lifetime away, more like a dream compared to this all-too-real doctor's visit. Whenever I was there, my eyes always wandered to a strange, framed drawing Dr. Russin had hung on the wall. It depicted another doctor's office, with a waiting room not unlike hers, but all of the patients in the picture were animals. The lion had a thermometer in his mouth. The crocodile's tail was in a cast. The doctor was nowhere in sight, but I always wondered if she was an animal, too.

It had been almost six months since the aneurysm's rupture, and Dr. Russin informed me it was time to schedule the routine post-operative angiogram. Consider this a progress report, she said.

I wasn't concerned much about my treated aneurysm. My language was improving, and every neurological and therapeutic expert I consulted seemed satisfied with my progress. My own personal gauge was probably centered around my journal. I felt the entries had become more detailed, more precise. Furthermore, I no longer needed it as a tool to communicate with others; instead, it had become a source of deep personal satisfaction, a forum where I could explore my thoughts, impressions, and daily inquiries.

It provided an outlet for expression that conversation with other people never seemed to accommodate.

However, I was a little confused about what an angiogram was, and asked Dr. Russin if she could break it down for me.

It's just a scan, she said. A somewhat invasive scan. She explained that a small incision would be made near the groin, and a camera would be snaked up through the body through a surgical catheter, much like my procedure in Scotland. Once the team could observe the aneurysm up close, they would inspect the coils and make sure they were still blocking off the blood flow from the rest of the brain. There would be an operating team in the room, ready to go if more support was needed.

It was as simple as that: a scan could become a surgery. The information felt like a stiff smack that left its stinging imprint on me long after the momentary action. I had assumed surgery was out of the question at that moment, but the possibility didn't faze Dr. Russin in the slightest. I was a little embarrassed to be so misinformed. It was my lack of knowledge, the limits of my own foresight, that had left me exposed in this way. This stung most of all.

And what about the second aneurysm? I asked her, a bit tentatively.

Dr. Russin said the procedure was only focused on the primary aneurysm, since it was the larger one, and because it needed to be checked up on more often. The secondary aneurysm was just something we had to be aware of.

Primary and secondary aneurysms—I had a mined mind. Whether I was having a scan or a surgery next month, this was the sort of thing I'd like to avoid in the future.

How long have I had these aneurysms? And what exactly caused them? I asked.

It is hard to say that with certainty, she said. Family history can be a factor. Hypertension, too. Cigarette use. Do you fall into any of those risk categories?

No, I said. I don't think so.

Well, this is where things get a little less clear. Babies usually don't get brain scans so there is no widespread way of checking, but it's possible that lots of people with aneurysms are just born with them.

Born with them. That was an entirely new concept for me to consider. Before the stroke, I had been active, ate a disproportionate amount of kale and very little meat. I practiced yoga nearly daily, before and after the rupture. Still, I knew that the aneurysm could not have been completely random, so there were probable causes. There were the small doses of steroids in the prescriptions I had been taking since I was a child to combat my asthma. I had been taking birth control since I was a teenager, and liberally sampled an assortment of illegal drugs as an undergraduate. I had made peace with the idea that any of those decisions had led to an aneurysm's formation. But this was the very first time it occurred to me that they might have simply been inevitable. Their threat could be as old as I was. If these aneurysms had grown up inside and alongside me, was the rest of my mind aware of these parts of my brain? Had my brain communicated that knowledge to my body? Had a subconscious knowledge of this been shaping my identity my whole life? A quiet preparation of things that would come to pass. And had the date and time of the rupture been predetermined? Was it always scheduled to happen the night of August 23, 2007—wherever I was, whatever I was doing? If a large aneurysm was bound to form—and bound to rupture—the most formative event of my life had nothing to do with the decisions I had personally made.

When I was at NYU, I had pursued a minor in religious studies. This meant my backpack was often weighed down with the writings of Sufi mystics, or rabbinical examinations pulled from the midrash. On my daily subway commute to school, I would pass a mosaic at the Lorimer Street stop, a rendering of a boulder balancing precariously, like a golf ball resting on a tee. There were two words on opposing sides of this giant rock: "Faith" and "Fate." I was an American, white, and born into an upwardly mobile, middle-class family. I had never felt especially oppressed by the idea of destiny, but the artwork reminded me of a spiritual question posed throughout human history: How much of a person's life depends on what they did, and how much of it is what is done to them? Now, this was something I couldn't get out of my mind.

Dr. Russin was ready to conclude our exam and clutched her clipboard to her chest. Well, Lauren? Are there any other questions I can answer for you?

Of course there weren't; that was the problem. We were completely in the realm of the unanswerable at that point. I was just being reminded of the terrifying knowledge we all innately understand, but do our best to ignore: there are forces inside of us that we can neither prevent nor control. And once I looked down into this well in myself, the drop seemed to go on forever.

17

My dad was driving me to speech therapy and quizzing me on today's subject: words with multiple meanings. I loved homophones and homonyms. It was comical that some *steaks* could be made of beef, and people gambled with *stakes*. *Toast* was a plain breakfast food as a noun, but as a verb, you could arrange a huge celebration and *toast* an appointed person.

Yeah, he said. *Toast* can be pretty tricky. And if you're not careful, you'll just find yourself in a *jam*.

I groaned.

Wow, he said. Tough crowd.

We were thoroughly enjoying this time together, and he told me that it reminded him of our interactions when I was very young, learning these words for the first time. He used to tease me, he said, when he would buckle me into my car seat. I'd start to smash my grubby toddler digits against the car window, and he'd make this defeated expression and say, *Poor window. Sad window.* And because I didn't know better, I would always ask him how he knew the window was sad.

It was meant to be a kind of call and response, my dad said. I would tell you that the window was suffering and you should be able to know that by feeling it.

Feeling what? I asked him. The window's pane?

Exactly! My dad slapped his thigh. It's pain! Oof. That never gets old.

And then the point of the joke dawned on me all over again.

Language sometimes needs a slow release, my dad said. You just have to grow into it.

He instructed me to make sure that Justine and Alicia talked to me about autoantonyms as well, words or phrases you can only know by their context, because one meaning could directly contradict the other. Like *trimming the tree* can mean cutting down its boughs or decking them in tinsel. You can *cleave* meat apart, but people cleave together.

Or *fight with*? I asked my dad. Because you can fight with someone on opposing sides, but you can also fight with someone as a combined force. On the same team.

That's my clever girl, my dad said, tousling my hair. Laura is going to be so impressed when she sees you next week.

Laura was traveling from New York to visit her parents in Northern California, and they were planning to swing through LA to see my parents and me. I was excited for the visit, but I had just gotten back from seeing Jonah in Seattle, and I had seen Grace in December. It felt like more than enough socializing for a while. I wanted to spend some time on my own. When I explained this to my dad, his lips formed a straight line, and he paused before responding.

You know, your friends have been missing you, kiddo. You've got to appreciate that. And actually, it seems to me that things were a little . . . tense . . . after you and Grace saw each other.

It turned out fine, I said. Not a big deal.

Maybe not a big deal for you, my dad said. But what about her? Have you asked her? I'm not going to push this point too hard, but I want you to remember that Grace has done a lot for you. All of your friends have. When you had to leave your PhD program, Grace spoke to all the administrators and your teachers on your behalf. She set everything in place for when you go back.

If I go back, I corrected him.

If. When. Whatever. You'll decide that when the time comes, he said. But friendship is a give and take. And you've been taking a little more than giving these days. People understand that that's the natural order of things. But try to appreciate all this from your friends' perspectives.

I knew it was something I had to work on.

Okay, Pop, I said. I'll try.

Laura couldn't stay in LA for long. She wouldn't even be in the state when I was going to have my angiogram in two weeks. But she did want to see me while she was on the West Coast. She and her parents drove down from the Bay Area to visit family in Long Beach. And while they were in town, my mother insisted on taking them out to lunch, choosing a restaurant directly across the street from Pasadena City Hall.

Our families sat together in the courtyard of a café that used to be a chapel. Our table was nestled against a brick wall, and the afternoon sun was coming through the stained glass.

If you don't mind, my mom said, tapping on her water glass with her spoon. I'd like to toast Laura, who was such a great help and comfort to Tony and me when we first arrived in Scotland. Valerie and Jim, you've raised an incredible young woman. I would hate to think about what could have happened if Laura hadn't been with Lauren that terrifying night back in August.

My dad interrupted the toast with a very loud hiccup. Since I was sitting beside him, I felt the jerk of his chair hitting mine. I expected a second hiccup, but instead, there was a low groan. *MMMMMNNNN.* I asked him if he was okay, but he didn't immediately respond. The sound behind his closed lips increased and became more strained. My mother started asking him questions that he also seemed unable to answer, and we both leaped up, fearing the worst: choking, heart attack, stroke. In another moment or two, my dad became aware that our physical concern for him was at an all-time high.

His lips finally loosened. You can sit back down, he said to us. I bit my cheek.

Your *cheek*? I asked incredulously. Are you kidding me? You just *bit* your *cheek*?

Oh, for Pete's sake, Tony, Mom said with mild annoyance, returning to her place at the table. Such theatrics.

What do you mean, Suzanne? It's not like I was overreacting, he said. It really *hurts*.

Looking to the other side of the table, it was clear to me Laura's family had been as concerned as we had been. Her father looked positively stricken. His face was as white as the table linen, his eyes still wide in horror.

Dad, you see Jim's expression over there? I said, motioning across the table. That is a "disaster" expression if I ever saw one.

My mother and I apologized, both to Laura's family and to neighboring tables, where concerned customers had taken out their cell phones, ready to call emergency services on our behalf. My father looked a little chagrined, but even in his sheepishness he appeared to be enjoying being the center of attention a little.

After the false alarm, the nervous energy at the table quickly transformed into total amusement. Laura and I found it impossible to restrain our giggles.

When I spoke to BJ on the phone a day or two later, I recounted that afternoon, complaining about my father's behavior.

That's interesting, BJ said. I remember when I first saw you with your folks many years ago. I couldn't totally understand your family dynamic. Actually, I thought you sort of condescended to your dad, and I was just flabbergasted by the way Californians spoke to their parents.

Oh, come on, I said. How did this become about Californian families all of a sudden?

We are products of our environment, Lauren, BJ said. You know that. All Texans have some cowboy, redneck streak in them, and all Californians can't help being a little hippie-weirdo sometimes. Your dad and your brother have their extreme personalities, with their high highs and their low lows. But your whole family unit works really well, especially when you or your mom function as the neutralizing forces, keeping them in check. And your whole aneurysm debacle must have upset this balance of power in a lot of ways.

Huh, I said. You might be on to something there. . . .

After all, there had been that violent incident over my brother's birthday, and soon after that, my mother being hospitalized. I couldn't remember what "normal" was but was sure this was not it. This might just be what it looked like when my family members were thrown out of their natural orbit.

I'm almost tempted to ascribe some significance to this hiccupping interlude, BJ said. Your dad playing the fool at lunch, and you and your mom putting him in line afterward? Sounds like you guys are being slowly nudged back to your original roles. Restoring the instinctive order of the play.

18

The street noise outside Jonah's Brooklyn bedroom window crackled through the phone, making it difficult to hear him. He had wanted to read the essay I had sent to Grace. I had taken her notes into serious consideration and made several changes before I sent it to him, hoping to emphasize my gratitude much more, while still highlighting the strange way language was influencing my entire worldview.

But things had taken a vexing turn, almost right away.

I think your sense of causality is all mixed up in here, Jonah said. And like Grace had done before him, he started to reference and cite the essay specifically, reading my text aloud to me:

Words breed dread. I know. As an adult, learning language again, I am sure of it. Images accompanying phrases readily, as if it is the first time. Utter the word 'nightmares,' makes the nightmares appear. It was only after I left the hospital with my parents when I began to know fear again, absorbing their own world of words. Misgiving. Rupture. Relapse. These words inscribed fear in a new heart.

Jonah stopped.

Right there, he said. You make it seem as if words were the problem. And that just can't be true. Words are symbols, not agents. They don't make things *appear*, they describe things that *are*. Language represents problems that exist, with or without words.

It's more complicated than that, Jo, I said.

I tried to explain how language could have a strange summoning effect, like the idea of the semantic tree and its severed branches. When I pinpointed an exact word or a phrase, a swarm of memories and images could sometimes come with it, and they were not always welcome. It felt that words made something appear that didn't exist without them. I was irritated that Jonah was calling my own experience a misrepresentation, since he had no basis for comparison.

Okay, okay, Jonah said. This doesn't have to be a debate about ontology. There are personal issues at stake for me, too. You just talk about everyone around you as a group, and I wanted to think of myself as a much more individual force throughout your recovery. This essay made me think that I was never that important to you.

Why would you think that? I asked.

I told him I hadn't been writing about him, specifically, but he felt I must've been, reminding me that he called all the time, and during the period I wrote the bulk of the essay, we spoke every day.

We did? I asked.

We *do*. We still do, Lauren. That's what I mean. Jesus, am I just wasting my breath here?

I heard him slam his bedroom window shut, its weatherized frame rattling upon impact.

I'm sorry if I'm overreacting, he said. It's never an easy transition from the glory of Seattle to the filth of Brooklyn. There's not enough space, and it's way too loud. I'm considering a move. I don't just want a bedroom for sleeping and a kitchen for eating. I want a living room for, you know, *living*. Because I might not always want to live alone forever.

You're considering a roommate again? I asked, honestly interested.

Not exactly, Jonah said. But I'd certainly like to be able to have company. Like you, for instance.

I told Jonah I didn't know when a trip like that would happen. On the obvious level, there was the uncertainty of the brain scan. But other than that, things were going pretty well in LA and if I flew to New York, I'd have to figure out my school situation, living situation, job situation. Would I have to reach out to the subletter in my apartment and ask her if I could stay there too? There was just a world of expectations waiting to crush me the second I arrived in the city.

Honey, Jonah said, as far as New York is concerned, you don't have to do anything, go anywhere, or see anybody. You don't even have to go to your apartment, if you don't want to.

I understood then that he was inviting me to stay in his place the whole time. I had never slept in Jonah's apartment for longer than a two-day stretch. It felt like a bit of a perilous situation. Though I was drawn to the idea of spending this time with him, we had no precedent for real cohabitation. What if I arrived, and soon after he decided he didn't want me there? Or what if I wanted out myself, but I had no bed to sleep in? It just might go terribly wrong.

Jonah, I only have enough money for groceries and subways. If you want us to be roommates, how would that work? Split the rent? Or should I divide my time in BJ's and Laura's apartments too?

You are making a mountain out of a molehill, Jonah teased, trying to ease my concern. I've got a place. I'm offering to have you stay in this place. Just come. That's all you have to do. Come. Stay.

I didn't feel like I could mention this to Jonah, but I couldn't stop fixating on the word *stay*. Stay. In my journals, I wondered: What does this mean? It reminded me of something people said to dogs. *Sit*. Good dog. *Stay*.

talking to me about a plans for a new apartment. come, stay with me.
The p words so easily expressed, the care behind them—I feel alienated.
COMe (Leave where you are)

Stay (here in ~~the~~ New York a new world of expectations) <u>Stay</u>. Dog sit.
How long would I stay?
With Me: Don't I have a home in NY? ~~Don~~ I did. ~~With~~ a sublettor is in
my bed right now. Live in his place, stay in his house, come from where I
am to meet him. And with me? ~~The new~~ Who is he to me? ~~Who~~ A friend,
a boyfriend, a housemate.
No one is safe. No one is comforting. No one is desired.

I'll never be able to account for all of the small moments of friction that my language disorder created between Jonah and me. I was sure that my aphasia was affecting not only my ways of perceiving the world, but also how I analyzed and reported on these perceptions.

This idea of *linguistic relativity* has always been a contentious one, sparking debates for years, across disciplines. It is sometimes referred to as the *Sapir-Whorf Hypothesis*. Sapir and Whorf were linguists who conducted most of their research at the beginning of the twentieth century, although they never even coauthored a paper together, let alone a hypothesis. Still, both men believed in a strong interdependence between language and thought, and the statements put forth in Whorf's book *Language, Thought, and Reality* were extremely bold. He wrote, "Language is not merely a reproducing instrument for voicing ideas but rather is itself the shaper of ideas." He went on to suggest that language molded aspects of our personal experiences, but moreover, it also formed our very abilities to *perceive* those experiences. And these ideas enthralled generations to come.

This hypothesis in its purest form fell out of favor because, in spite of Whorf's claims of doing "unbiased research" standing on "unimpeachable evidence," current (and appropriate) criticisms of Whorf usually address his amateurism and cultural plundering.

However, Sapir and Whorf shaped the debate about the power of language in the mind, and their influence is still very much felt—with a lot of renewed interest in linguistic relativity—in more nuanced forms. But there is significant resistance to it from camps who are more invested in Universal Grammar, and hoping to understand the "language organ." As Steven Pinker contends, "The idea that thought is the same thing as language is an example of . . . a conventional absurdity," adding, "If thoughts depended on words, how could a new word ever be coined?" And this was part of the position Jonah was representing. Words were always symbols, never agents—they could only have a very limited scope in the thought process because they had no inherent powers of creation themselves.

At this point, I can see the virtues of all sides of this incredibly complex language debate, and my allegiances aren't entirely fixed anymore. But at the time, language was still being rekindled in me, and I was resentful that Jonah was ignoring my unique authority on language relativity. I was the one with a linguistic disorder—what were his qualifications to prove me wrong?

Still, it's hard not to wonder how radically different Jonah's recollections of this exact same conversation might be.

We all know firsthand how our memories differ from person to person, even if we were side by side in the events being recalled. But we rarely think about the ways new experiences can actually affect our abilities to remember the old ones. Nonetheless, a memory changes every time we remember it. Or as Daniel Schacter writes in *The Seven Sins of Memory*, "It is difficult to separate . . . 'the way we were' from current appraisals of 'the way we are.'"

There are so many frailties intrinsic to both language and memory, and how attached we become to our personal narratives. We tell ourselves that we are certain types of people. And to maintain consistency in our own recollections, and to avoid the pain of cognitive dissonance, we justify and accommodate our memories. We trim and exaggerate. And the vast majority of the time, we do all of this without even realizing it. In this way, it's hard to imagine what is actually mutual in this life, and whether two different people can ever be on the same journey together.

The first vacation Jonah and I ever took was early in our relationship. We made an impromptu trip to upstate New York for a weekend so we could visit a sculpture garden called Storm King. We had no car and no place to stay. When we arrived, we discovered that almost all the hotels were closed for the season, and the same for the outdoor museum. But we were invigorated by that challenge. We convinced an owner of an officially "closed" bed and breakfast that we were newlyweds, so he let us stay that night. At Storm King, we snuck in, leaping over creeks and fallen trees, making it our personal playground. We kissed against the weathered iron, plunged our hands into each other's jeans, keeping an eye out for the guard on patrol. Spontaneous, inventive, irreverent—this was us at our best.

Our next major adventure, however, was completely different. A year later, Jonah was admitted into a summer program in Amsterdam, a coveted and competitive appointment among the acting students at NYU. Perhaps more well-known than the program's prestige was the havoc it wreaked on relationships. These were young actors at the height of their physical peak, in sweltering weather, rehearsing in little to no clothing in a city where drugs were legalized . . . it wasn't very conducive to fidelity. If one member of a couple went to Amsterdam while the other stayed behind, it usually meant the death of their romance. Very few couples remained unscathed after one of its members "went Dutch."

Before our impending separation, Jonah made it clear he had no intention of letting our relationship dissolve this way. He made all sorts of overtures in the form of dates and gifts, and once, when I had left him alone at my house, he even slipped a note between my pillows, a prose poem of sorts—*Lauren Marks. Marks, I you. You, I Marks. You Lauren, you Marks, love. Love I. I love. You love. I love you Lauren Marks.*

After he left for Amsterdam, he continued to be clear about his persistent feelings. If he was tempted by the sensual nature of Amsterdam, he didn't act on it. Instead, he incurred exorbitant fees calling me in New York a few times a week. He soon hatched the idea that I should meet him in Europe when his program finished. This wasn't that easy. Jonah could still rely on his father's financial contributions until his graduation, but I was spending the summer scrounging for babysitting and tutoring gigs. Luckily, being a performer in New York had taught me to live on the cheap. By combining our limited resources, including a gift of his father's frequent flyer miles, we made the trip happen.

Our European sojourn started with a blissful reunion. In Switzerland and Italy, we stayed with some friends from NYU, sharing car rides and tiny hotel rooms, bohemian-style. But soon I was reminded how quickly the barometric pressure could change with Jonah. When a mood struck him, a sort of funnel cloud would form. No desire tempted, no words comforted. Everything and everyone was temporarily obliterated by the howling tempest whistling off his skin. It was a void that I could not bargain with.

In the picturesque villages of Cinque Terre, we wandered away from our friends for a few hours, walking the beach beneath a starless sky. Jonah started to bitterly complain. He had been waiting for me to join him in Europe, pining and planning, and for what? This was not at all the trip he had bargained for. I can't remember if he directly accused me of being responsible for his current dissatisfaction, but my vulnerable mind started to spin it like that. Our problems, real and imaginary, were suddenly numbering in the thousands. And I felt hopelessly implicated in every single one.

I may or may not have voiced that sense of dread to Jonah, but I let the tears burn down my face, drying in the hot Mediterranean breeze. We had not reconciled when we returned to the cramped, single room we shared with that other couple. I had hoped his abject mood would lift the next morning, but he had stopped speaking to me entirely by the time we'd boarded the overnight train to Rome. As the sun rose the next morning, we were near the Colosseum and our suitcases were rattling over the broken cobblestones. Our plan had been no plan. What had been so charming and exciting in upstate New York felt desperate in Italy. I scoured the streets for any place to stop.

I dashed toward the first hotel that looked open. It was small and a little run-down, but being picky wasn't an option. I handed over my credit card without even asking for the price. These mood swings in Jonah weren't very common, and whenever they began at home, I would just go back to my own apartment, something I couldn't do here. I thought if we could just lie down together, we could sleep it off and wake up refreshed and relaxed. In the room, I reached toward Jonah and tried to direct him to the bed. With a rough sweep, he just brushed my hand aside and headed toward the shower.

While he turned on the water, I took a bleak inventory. A bed. A bureau. A few hangers. What was I supposed to do in this room without him?

The unframed mirrors in the bedroom had a reflective trigonometry, making it possible to see into the bathroom mirrors without even facing them. Jonah had left the door open and I watched his shape distort through the shower's dappled glass. He was a mass of intolerable blurriness. I resented Jonah's indifference to me, then resented resenting it. Why had I ever agreed to this trip when there was clearly no escaping it?

Then? *Out.* Out was the only way.

There were locations in the world where I was still wanted, maybe even needed, and I had to return to a place where I felt necessary again. The practical considerations began to whir, though. It was a nonrefundable ticket—how would I pay to get back to New York?

But I muzzled the nagging doubt. I could handle a little credit card debt if I had to. And though it was going to be embarrassing to explain to BJ and Laura why I had to return so early, they wouldn't make a bad situation worse. I zipped my suitcase and rolled it to the door.

And then Jonah stepped into the room in a towel, slippery as a newborn.

Was he feeling better? Or was it an illusion produced by the red heat rising from his skin?

What are you doing? Jonah asked.

I'm . . . I hesitated. I'm leaving, I said finally. I'm going home. I tightened my grip on my bag to show him I was serious—and to steady myself, too. Really don't know what happened here or how I can change it, I continued. And I'm not saying it's your fault, Jo. But I can't stay with this . . . nothingness . . . between us.

Jonah stood exactly where he was. So I unlocked the door to let myself out.

Don't, he said, so quietly I could hardly hear him. Don't go.

I think I have to, I said. How can I stay with things like this?

Well, you shouldn't have to leave. Still, he said, I can't give you a good reason to stay, either.

This was our impasse. Neither one of us wanted to linger in despair, neither wanted a fight or an extravagant exit. There seemed no sensible course of action available, until my nervous fingers encountered a coin in my pocket.

Should we leave it to fate? I asked him, taking out the coin. Heads, I stay, tails, I leave.

There was a long pause from Jonah, while the water pooled on the wood floor where he was standing. Then he nodded.

When reason is exhausted, he said, there is only the unreasonable to explore.

I tossed the coin.

It glinted as it soared and twisted in the air on an unusually long flight, as if conscious of the weight of its own mediation. When it glided down to the bed, I released my grip on the suitcase and Jonah tightened his towel. Both of us stepped forward to read the verdict.

Heads.

With no hesitation at all, we clutched at each other, our bodies becoming a tangle on top of the fateful coin. We didn't apologize because there was nothing and everything to forgive. The situation was beyond our reckoning, composed of aspects far beyond our own invention. It felt our union was being sanctified by luck itself.

Stay with me? he pleaded.

Stay, stay, he said. So I stayed.

19

It was February before I considered Justine's idea that learning sign language might be helpful to my recovery. I hadn't initially been able to follow her advice because my workload with her had been too demanding, but as soon as I thought I would be able to manage it, my mother found a course for me at the Greater Los Angeles Agency on Deafness (GLAD). It was even close enough to my parents' house for me to drive myself to class.

The GLAD building was old Los Angeles chic—red tile roof, wrought-iron fire escapes, and an open, green courtyard. I arrived a bit early to find the front door unlocked. As I wandered through the hallways, the carpeted floor muffled my footsteps. But where was everyone? Had I come on the wrong day? I was still easily confused by dates and times. More self-conscious with every step, I tiptoed by the bathrooms and the drinking fountains, and when I spied a sign that read "cafeteria," I followed it.

When I looked through the cafeteria window, I was surprised to see about thirty people and a party underway. They were milling around, pouring themselves coffee and snatching donuts from open boxes. Their necks craned and their hands were animated in what appeared to be lively exchanges. The door between the action and me was thin, but I couldn't hear any sounds from inside. It was as if I were peering from a porthole in a submarine, observing the animated life of the busy sea. I was mesmerized by so much conversation conducted so silently. I easily figured this wasn't my class, but I knew I was in the right place.

The activity started to wind down, and others began to gather at the door with me. Then, our teacher, Sarahlena, a cute blonde with cork-screw curls and blue jeans, strolled past. She indicated that we should enter the room now. Two things became instantly clear to all of us: first, Sarahlena was deaf, and second, she could read lips extremely well. With students consisting of exclusively hearing people, this talent was incredibly useful.

The first day was full of fumbling. She passed around worksheets with the American Sign Language alphabet, instructing the class to try asking and answering questions while practicing their fingerspelling. She communicated by writing on the blackboard, though all of us struggled with her rule of not asking questions aloud, especially with her back turned. The protocol made perfect sense, but took a little getting used to.

What is your name? Sarahlena wrote on the board.

The students clumsily tried to sign their answers, but everyone had to consult their handouts. None of us knew the ASL alphabet yet, so our hands stuttered. Still, it was exciting to be in the company of other people who were so actively struggling with their words. In this unique environment, it was like all of us were suffering from the same language disorder.

For the second round of questions, Sarahlena wrote on the blackboard: *What brought you to this class? Why do you want to learn ASL?*

Everyone had a different reason. One person fingerspelled W-E-D-D-I-N-G. Another, S-O-N. Sarahlena seemed to understand people's answers, though we students had a much harder time following one another. We all kept looking down at our alphabets, and every time we broke eye contact, we'd lose our place in the conversation.

Then it was my turn.

I fingerspelled: A-N-E-U-R-Y-S-M.

Sarahlena looked at me quizzically.

My new teacher repeated my word back, with a question lingering on her hands: A-N-E-U-R-Y-S-M?

Yes. I nodded. B-R-A-I-N aneurysm. I pointed to myself. A-P-H-A-S-I-A.

This was not something I usually shared in public because I didn't want the attention it might bring. But I knew that everyone else was equally inexperienced with this fingerspelling, and it was entirely possible that only my teacher understood my disclosure. It was our secret.

The first ASL lesson had all the basics of any language class: how to answer yes or no questions, how to explain when you didn't understand. In sign language, I discovered that there weren't different words for *scared*, *terrified*, *alarmed*, and *panicked*. They shared the exact same sign, but it could be expressed at different levels of physical intensity. In spoken language, I still struggled with synonyms. It was laborious to learn twelve words meaning the same thing, and then be expected to refine the perfect usage and context for each one. With sign language, one word would do as long as you expressed it well.

Sarahlena insisted that everyone in the class had to be much more demonstrative. They had to drop their neutral expression, and the propriety associated with personal boundaries. How rigid were your hands? How wide were your eyes? All were integral parts of employing this language.

When your face is vacant, so are your words, Sarahlena explained. Your face changes your meaning entirely in ASL. It can be the difference between a conflict and a joke. She put a supremely goofy expression on her face. It is okay to be S-I-L-L-Y, she signed and spelled. Just never be B-L-A-N-D.

At GLAD, I was starting to understand that language and gesture had a lot in common. Being immersed in so much physical imitation seemed to shape, or at least sharpen, some of my language skills. In the hospital five months earlier, I wouldn't have been able to remember or recite my traditional alphabet. But now, when Justine asked me to go through the alphabet, I could do one aloud and another on my hands. I wasn't even consulting my notes. This was proof that my attention span had gotten stronger and I could learn and memorize more.

I'm not even the worst student in the class! I beamed at Justine. Everyone around me is struggling too.

Have you been able to continue your reading? she asked.

I'm taking a break from the long Casanova memoir, but started a much shorter book: the autobiography of Helen Keller.

Was that an assignment for your ASL class? she asked.

No, it was my mom's copy. When she was a teenager, she played Helen Keller in a production of *The Miracle Worker*.

I told Justine how interesting I found the phrases Keller chose to employ in her text. She wrote "I saw" and "I heard" a lot, even though she couldn't do either. And the supplementary materials to her book were just as good. It wasn't just Helen telling her story to a wide readership years later; the writings of her teacher, Anne Sullivan, were included too. Helen had even permeated my dreams.

The Sullivan letters are incredible, I explained. Sometimes you can find a letter that will correspond with something Keller has recounted in her book, but the Sullivan document was written on the day the events actually transpired. So it's the difference between real-time reporting and hind . . . oh . . . umm . . . hindmind?

Hind*sight*.

Yes, I said. Exactly. The difference between real-time reporting and hindsight. These two types of writing can be so radically different from each other. I love those layers.

That's so cool! Justine said, an oversize grin on her face. It was thoroughly enjoyable to share this information with someone who seemed equally invested. See you this time next week? she asked.

But I couldn't immediately respond. My mother had told me that our insurance company was threatening to stop covering my sessions. She had left them a couple of messages and we were waiting to hear back from them. I had avoided mentioning it earlier because speech therapy was my home away from home, and I had hoped I could continue with my sessions as usual.

Reluctantly, I decided that there was no time like the present, and explained the situation. Justine wasn't at all surprised.

It was bound to happen, she lamented. It's criminal if you ask me, but speech therapy is usually only subsidized for the first few months after a stroke. We will figure this out together.

We will? I asked. How?

Don't know yet, she said. If you can't pay for sessions anymore, maybe we could do bartering for a little while—a sort of therapy exchange? Might be able to use your talents in helping out another patient of mine.

Um, I murmured. Maybe, but I am not sure how I could be helpful. . . .

Justine nodded. Let me think about it and get back to you, she said.

Soon after the suggestion that I might be placed in some kind of a position of authority again, I went on to dream vividly of Helen Keller and Casanova, where my subconscious spared no expense in displaying my carnival of insecurities.

Dream

LOCATION: huge empty warehouse

I am friends with Cassanova and ~~whe~~ suggests an activity, a display. We were to <u>reconvene</u> after we had a time to show what we had been working on (<u>auto-biographical</u>?)

Cassanova went first. He ~~m~~had spent a great deal of money and props. The audience consisted of only two people, me and Helen Keller. His project fills the whole warehouse. He conjured up a ~~gaggle~~ galling of figures. Living and dead, physical and ethereal, spanning incredible ages of time. The lights of dead flickering like phosphourescents in the sea.

It was my turn. I used the empty space and used my own body. I began to fly, I inch, a gesture, I contort. There was a sense Cassanova and Keller were not as impressed.

*I thought his piece was incredible but hardly plausibly autobiographical
but slick. He had felt mine was not slick enough, lacking necessary
artifice. She didn't say, but Keller seemed to be on his side.*

A few days after our session, Justine clarified what she meant by a "therapy
exchange," telling me she had arranged for me to meet another client of
hers. I nervously warmed to the idea.

This tutoring was just a one-time thing, she said, something we would
experiment with and discuss afterward. The young woman attended speech
and language therapy, too, though our sessions took place on different days,
so our paths hadn't crossed before. Justine explained that the girl was working on admission requirements for high school applications, and she was
starting a personal essay.

But why do you think I could help her? I asked, unsure.

Why not? Justine said. Essays are much more your specialty than mine
these days.

Alicia and Justine cleared off a small desk for me in between their of-
fices. It wasn't a proper room, just part of the hallway in an alcove with the
fax machine, but it could serve the purpose well enough. The girl, Chloe,
arrived without the clamor I expected from a teenager. Clear-eyed, she
stood in the corridor silent and slim as a birch tree, with an unusually
graceful bearing.

Take a seat, I said, introducing myself in my most professional voice.
Justine tells me you are applying to high schools?

Chloe's long hair fell into her face and she placed the errant strands
behind her ear as she sat down.

A couple of schools, yeah, she said. The wood surface between us had
just enough room for two sets of hands, so when she pulled out her note-
book, she kept it on her lap.

Have you written down something already? I asked. Can I see it?

It's just scribbling, she said, gripping the folder tightly. I thought I
should write about dance. Or maybe what I do in student council. I think I

am supposed to tell them something important about me, but I can't think of anything big. My life is pretty boring.

I seriously doubt that, I said, trying to impersonate someone who knew what she was doing.

What advice could I give as a writing tutor? Aside from my time at GLAD, I still hadn't really revealed my language condition in public. Still, I could write about my aphasia in my journals and explore it in an essay. I knew I could admit things in my writing that I would never say aloud. I couldn't remember my high school application process, but I suspected that at this age a lot of applicants tended to sound alike.

Everyone writes what they think a selection committee wants to hear, I said. They write about all their accomplishments, what they want to do after college, and all their big plans. But no one really knows what they are doing yet. I'd much rather hear about something you don't want your new school to know about you.

The girl's eyes looked pained. What do you mean?

I told her that vulnerability, and expressing that vulnerability well, can differentiate a person from the pack in a very striking way.

She gave a sidelong look at the fax machine, and started to absentmindedly pick at her fingernail polish. My tenuous confidence was instantly deflated—I had lost her. This approach had been my only big idea for her essay, and it appeared to be falling flat, perhaps making her too embarrassed to continue. Did the girl think I was employed in this practice? Or had Justine already told her that I was a patient too? Either way, I was sure my incompetence had been unmasked.

Well . . . the girl said tentatively. And my ears quickly perked up.

Yeah? I asked.

I . . . I suck my thumb, she said. My whole life, and even now sometimes, when I'm nervous. That's why I lisp. That's why I came to speech therapy in the first place.

I hadn't heard any lisp at all, but I was overjoyed by her prospective topic. That's exactly what you should include on your application! I exclaimed.

The girl's shoulders locked together. No, she said. No way. That's, like, a kindergartener problem. No self-respecting school would accept me after I told them that.

We never want to admit weakness, I said. But our weaknesses can define us much more than our strengths. They aren't always bad things to have.

She looked at me, somewhat confused, and I didn't blame her. Before the rupture, this idea of strength in weakness wouldn't have made much sense to me, either. I realized this was an opportunity, though. Not just for this girl, but for me, too. Only minutes earlier, I had relished the idea that this girl might mistake me as an experienced, neurotypical professional, but now I wanted her to see me as someone who was also actively struggling with my speech, not so different from her at all.

My parents like to remind me that I had an early predisposition toward language. Precocious by first grade, I was memorizing scenes from movies and TV shows, reciting back dialogue long before I could actually comprehend the meaning of the lines or understand whether the language was appropriate for a child or not. This youthful talent—and parents who owned an advertising agency—landed me a few commercials that ended up partially paying for my college tuition. As an actor, I delved into hundreds, if not thousands, of plays, committing many roles to memory. There were characters who spoke in riddles or songs, some in Elizabethan English, others in Dada garbles. At least once I had spoken all of my lines in a language I wasn't even fluent in. I had a long and luxurious romp in language, and when I was being trained at NYU, I let myself believe that I was well on my way to making a living in words. Still, this kind of passion required a "day job" to maintain. And by the time I became a grad student, overworked and underpaid, I didn't find nearly as much joy in words. Language subtly continued to affect my motivations, but the more experience I gained, the less I was aware of the ways it had shaped my landscape of desire. It had become a little ordinary.

After college, I faced the reality that a career in language rarely paid the rent. I still loved going onstage and still produced avant-garde pieces with my friends, but as my creativity thrived, my bank account did not. I didn't like to audition for shows I didn't care about, which meant I hardly auditioned at all. Five years after I had left college, I was reconsidering all of my life choices.

It was hard not to compare myself to my parents at my age. Not only had they found the person they would one day marry, they were working actors. They lived in Europe; my dad was writing plays, my mom was teaching children's theater, and they made extra money dubbing German movies into English. They were hardly rich, but they had pursued their passion for performance and lived off it. That was exactly what I wanted. So why hadn't I figured it out yet?

In this period of flux, I had applied to a couple of PhD programs and was accepted into a good one in New York. After my first year, I was awarded a full stipend for the next two terms, with a teaching fellowship. Soon, I would be leading a class of undergraduates in the speech department. Unlike my stalled artistic life, it felt like I was finally getting an appointment commensurate with some actual accomplishments.

This teaching position was one of the main reasons I decided to travel to see Krass in Paris in the first place; he had been one of my most influential instructors at university and I was hungry for guidance. Would my academic pursuits come at the expense of my life in art? I needed confirmation that this was the right path. I needed to know what I was doing, and how and why I was doing it. It had to be the right choice.

I remember the two of us sitting on his terrace, a white tablecloth between us, tea lights flickering. Krass peered into the globe of red wine in his hands as if he were examining tea leaves.

They will be lucky to have you, he said. I always knew you'd be a teacher.

But it didn't turn out that way at all. The day I should have started teaching "The Art of Public Speaking" in front of a college class in New York, I was in a hospital bed in Edinburgh unable to even say my parents' names.

Nonetheless, Krass's prediction was coming to pass, just not in a way I had ever expected. In Justine's speech therapy practice, I had no way of knowing if Chloe would follow my instructions—it was the first and last time I ever saw her. But it was clear that the advice I was giving her was something I needed for myself. I had told people that I was a writer even before I could finish a grammatical sentence. If I thought about that too much, there was something delusional about it, even fraudulent. That changed if I could dictate the terms, though. I started to let myself believe that I could be a writer *and* an aphasic, and that didn't have to be an oxymoron. Not really. Because people never excelled at anything until they had failed at it for a very, very long time.

20

A few nights later, Jonah and I were chatting over the phone. He was well aware that my go-to conversation topic these days tended to be Helen Keller, so he asked if I had encountered any new information about her that I found especially interesting.

Of course! I said. Did you know that the very first thing Helen published created a pretty big controversy? It even started a rift between her and her closest friends.

Don't think I ever heard about that, he said. What happened?

She was still a kid, really, I said. A short story she wrote was published, but soon after, people noticed that it had striking similarities to another story written by a different author. A contemporary. She had no memory of reading the story and didn't have a copy of it in her braille library. She sincerely thought the story was her own invention, but suddenly, she was under extreme scrutiny.

I explained that the most likely scenario was that the story had been signed into Helen's hand at some point and she had simply forgotten it happened. She was only twelve years old at the time, meaning she had only been using language for *four years*. This fable would've been coming to her alongside her history homework, her Latin, Greek, and French instructions, her rudimentary exposure to the life cycles of plants and animals. During that massive influx of new information in the form of words, someone probably signed the story, or some elements of the story, into her palm, making this quick transfer of nonessential material little more than an afterthought. But soon after she published the story under her name, she was forced to defend herself. Everything from her intelligence to her intention was called into question.

Wow, Jonah said. That's heavy.

It was hard for me to imagine how Helen created her systems of managing incoming information, sorting and prioritizing it. The field of her learning had been so parched, and then, all at once, it was drenched. It must have been so easy to misunderstand things as she was putting ideas into categories. I struggled with that sort of thing myself.

Can you imagine explaining copyright law to a twelve-year-old? I asked Jonah. Any twelve-year-old. Now, try to introduce the concept to a deaf child's hand. . . .

Uh-huh, Jonah said. His tone was a little distant.

Jonah?

Mmm.

Have you drifted off somewhere?

Jonah snapped back to attention. Oops, he said, flustered. Sorry.

No problem. I can get so absorbed in this stuff. What were you thinking about?

Forget it, he said. It was totally unrelated, and I promise it wouldn't at all further this discussion. Remind me what you were saying?

Oh, it's totally fine, I said. We can change the subject and discuss what's on your mind now. What is it?

Well, he said. If you must know . . .

And I must. I smiled into the phone. I must!

I was just thinking about sex, he said. With you, of course.

Now it was my turn to be flustered. I was always surprised when our conversations took a turn like this. It had been five and a half months since

Jonah and I lived in the same city, and my drive for physical intimacy had gone the way of my cravings for salty food or coffee or booze. My desires were inconstant and unfocused. It had been different when we had seen each other in person, but in general, I didn't have much mental space for longing.

It would've been hard to fault Jonah for being unable to remove sexuality from our dynamic, especially since it had been at the forefront of our past relationship. I had been flirtatious before the rupture, but I wasn't like that now. Jonah was torn between the demands and predilections of two entirely different women. Initially, he must have tried to please the woman he had known before her accident, and now he was learning to address her unfamiliar twin. The first woman wanted much more from him, and strangely, the second one wanted much less.

As I considered the sharp turn in this conversation, my own thoughts began to wander. I wondered specifically: How did Helen Keller deal with physical attraction? How did she perceive herself while she was being perceived?

The worldview Keller espoused in her book did not evoke the delicate body of the twenty-two-year-old who imagined its extensive philosophy. Keller was lithe and her unseeing eyes were bright and active. She was beautiful by even the most traditional standards. Propelled by her curiosity and formidable appetite for knowledge, she had attended Radcliffe University, and with Harvard a stone's throw away, she would have been constantly milling through the pulsing throngs of graduates and undergraduates, college students newly liberated from their parents' watchful gaze, their libidos significantly loosened. Was it possible that Keller had embarked on all of her passionate exertions without a single pheromone? Where was the space for the love of learning, the love of friends, and the love between lovers? How did they separate? When did they commingle? And how does one indulge in a single passion, without it being at the expense of all others? I just wanted Helen to advise me.

I had spent so much time physically separated from most of my social circle, and mainly disconnected from all things Internet. Yes, my reading was slow, but literature never rushed me. So my attachments to the people I read about in books were intensely personal. We were in a constant discussion, one in which I could never accidentally offend them. The way I read, and the way I used my journal, was taking up most of the space that used to be allotted for conversation with others. There was just less energy for dialogue with living, breathing beings who could be in the same room with me. This didn't mean that my need for that companionship totally went away, but it was safer for me to interact with characters in books than the people around me.

21

In mid-February, my final days of speech therapy and ASL classes at GLAD were both approaching. Although Justine and I had discussed the possibility of continuing our sessions, the financial difficulties couldn't be ignored.

If you really wanted to stay, Justine said, I could try to seek out more creative solutions. But, from my professional perspective, our classes have sort of developed into informal conversations instead of structured lessons.

And I actually agreed with her.

But I don't think I am done with my rehabilitation, I told her. Not even close. I certainly don't think I can go back to school or memorize lines for a play. So I don't know where to go from here.

Unfortunately, I can't tell you that either, she said. The goal of speech and language therapy after a stroke is to give patients the tools to be self-sufficient. And safe. You've been an unusual case from the very beginning.

What are the next steps for other people, usually? I asked her.

Most people who have had strokes aren't able to return to the exact life they had before, but I see you are motivated to do more work to hone your language skills. I certainly think you should proceed on your unique path, she said. But this is not the sort of thing I can help much with.

I'm just glad we were able to do it at all, I said. And I am relieved we finished a final draft of my essay before my angiogram.

It was my pleasure. But I am curious—what does that essay have to do with your upcoming procedure?

I thought this was self-explanatory.

Well, I said. Anything can change in a brain, right? So I want to have something written down. Finished. In case I wake up . . . different.

And "different" was a serious understatement. I wasn't stricken by fear exactly. It just felt like I was at the edge of something big, like a first-time skydiver, completely unsure what was on the other side of that jump. And brains changed. They just did. I felt I needed to put something out into the world before this brain changed on me again.

You know, I've thought about that essay a lot, Justine began. And I don't think your friends should have responded to it the way they did.

Oh no? I asked. I'm sort of glad they said what they said.

Having a support group is important, Justine said. And everyone is entitled to their personal opinions. Clearly they are very intelligent people and their love for you is abundant, which means a lot. I just wish they had been a little more understanding. . . .

I had felt the same way soon after I had spoken to Jonah and Grace. But my thoughts on the matter had evolved since then.

I think I need to be around people who really challenge me, I said. It's like medicine.

Sure, she said. Too much judgment can suffocate our growth or expression. But lack of judgment doesn't nourish us either.

Exactly, I said. Without them, it would've been impossible to put myself in context. I would have just continued to believe that everyone read my writing the same way I did. Which is a pretty limited idea. What would you call that? Neeve?

I looked for Justine's approval.

Naive, she said. And *naive* is the perfect word, Lauren. But there are worse things in the world than being naive.

22

I arrived at the USC hospital at the end of February for my six-month post-rupture angiogram. I was shown to a room, where I swiftly changed out of my yoga pants and into my hospital gown. A little restless, I waited for the doctor to arrive so we could get the whole thing over and done with. Instead, a woman dressed in a suit jacket and pants walked toward my room. Her gait was determined, almost strident. She looked at me cursorily, then at my parents, who were standing nearby. I had no idea who she was, or what she might want. She brandished a clipboard like a badge, and then asked, Who is financially responsible for this patient?

Money. It took a second to sink in. My sense of anxiety quickly transformed into irritation—these were moments of quiet reflection and preparation, to be spent with my family, mentally preparing myself for something entirely unknown. It felt completely inappropriate to discuss money right before this procedure began, and according to Laura and BJ, it had been radically different in Scotland. My friends had dutifully collected my passport and insurance cards when I was taken to the hospital and tried to deliver them to the appropriate entities, but no one was interested in such trivia. Some administrator told them that the doctors were busy trying to save their friend's life, and they would deal with these scraps of paper at a later date.

After my parents and the administrator worked out a payment plan, I was given a wristband and some forms to fill out. I tried to decode the abbreviations on the paperwork. Most of it was simple enough:

NME—Name

DOB—Date of Birth

ADD—Address

But the next one gave me pause: RLG.

RLG . . . I asked the woman. Is that asking about my religion?

Yes, she said. But if you don't identify with any traditional options, you can put "Other" if you'd like.

After a few moments of tense consideration, I left that line blank. I hadn't put *that* much thought into this trip to the hospital.

I was transferred from the bed to a gurney to a table in an operating room. Still alert and awake, my head was put into soft clamps. It felt like trying on a child's bike helmet. A heavy lead apron was draped on my torso, covering my feet and legs, and part of my hospital gown was peeled away at my upper right thigh. I could feel them shaving a small section around my upper groin, where the catheter would be inserted.

As powerful light bulbs were shifted to spotlight my body, the anesthesiologist appeared at my side. She was muscular and dark-skinned. Her voice was pleasant, as was her soothing touch against my arm. She looked for a place to insert the needle with as little pain for me as possible. I wouldn't feel anything, but I might be awake for the procedure.

This drug supports a *twilight sleep*, she said. You probably won't remember anything from this point on. Most people doze off before their angiograms begin.

The anesthesia kicked in quickly. Though I couldn't feel the nick near my groin, I did feel the jet of hot contrast dye that was inserted into the catheter and created a liquid stampede from my leg to my head. From that point on, I was too drugged for pain, only sensation. When the dye arrived at its intended target, the four blank screens to my left started to light up.

There was no way I could fall asleep now. The veins of my head began to sprout in front of me, like trees on an alien planet. It was surreal. I was both thinking and observing, realizing I was seeing the exact site of those thoughts and observations. I hadn't prepared to see all of this, though it didn't bother me. Everything around me was a psychotropic miracle. After a small bit of navigational chatter, I heard Dr. Teitelbaum speaking to his surgical team.

See that? he asked. Right over there?

And yes. They saw. Right there.

Well, looks like we can't do anything more today, he said conclusively.

His congress of colleagues easily agreed, but I didn't.

Why? I slurred. Why can't we do anything today?

Dr. Teitelbaum's eyes widened in shock, and his face mask billowed. He hadn't realized I was awake the whole time, clearly focused on the task at hand.

Are you quite comfortable down there, Lauren?

Better than comfortable, I said. S'brilliant. Greatest show on earth.

Would you like some more anesthetic? he asked. Because I am sure the anesthesiologist would be happy to give you a stronger dose.

No! I said. Don't change a thing. But whatssa problem, Doc?

The aneurysm at the middle cerebral artery has substantially recanalized, he said.

Oh. Mmm. I tried to mull this over, but my stupor didn't allow much high-level cognition. Recanny, I murmured. Recamping something. Say again?

He gave up trying to silence me. Think of a bag of potato chips, he said. From the outside, it looks like it's full, but when you open it up, the chips have all settled at the bottom.

I was far too high for metaphors. I was asking about my brain and Dr. Teitelbaum was discussing snack foods.

Can't you just put more coils into the aneurysm? I asked.

No. We can't, actually. The aneurysm is refilling with blood and its neck is too wide to keep coils in there. The shape just won't allow it. It looks like you're going to have to consider a craniotomy because that's the only way to treat this.

Oh, I said. Okay, then. Good. Well . . . I've considered it, I said. Go right ahead.

We can't do it now. Dr. Teitelbaum shook his head. The angiogram is a neuroradiological procedure that goes up a tube, but a craniotomy goes through the skull. That's not something I do. We have a surgeon in our practice who specializes in that, though. Dr. Giannotta.

All right, I said, trying to be as proactive as much as anyone on mind-altering drugs can be. You just get Dr. Digiorno and I'll wait right here.

Giannotta. And that's not possible today, Dr. Teitelbaum said, probably praying my jabbering would finally stop.

What about the other aneurysm? Can you do that one now? As long as you're up there?

It's in the other hemisphere. And it is too small to worry about at the moment, he answered. As far as the craniotomy is concerned, I'll try to arrange for Dr. Giannotta to see you right away. He could probably fit you in tomorrow.

The twenty-four hours between the angiogram and the craniotomy consult were strange, to say the least. When I was much more sober, I took in the actual dimensions of the thing. My head was going to be cracked open. It was an experience that people would spend their entire lives avoiding, but I would have to submit to it willingly and even have to pay for it! It was an uncomfortable idea to adjust to, and the absurdity of it brought me to the verge of tears and laughter simultaneously. But Dr. Teitelbaum said this was the only way to treat the aneurysm, so there didn't seem to be any other choice. I had to accept it quickly. However, with the little agency I had at my disposal, I started to think of the kind of language I could use in this surgical consult. Should I make a joke to relieve the tension a bit? Maybe I would tell the surgeon, "I'll give you a piece of my mind!"

More than anything, I felt I had to be practical, informed, and—even though I would struggle with this—completely stoic. I didn't want my prospective surgeon to see my weakness, because this whole operation was going to leave me exposed. I wanted to preserve my sense of dignity in some way. I wanted to exude hard-boiled grit. And I felt there might be someone who could actually help me get it.

The only thing I could think to do in way of preparation was to call my friend Shafer. A poet by day and bartender by night, he had been my drinking buddy for years. He indulged his life with a headlong gusto, and accordingly, he could be a reliable steward of just about any kind of conversation. He would discuss esoteric poetic forms like the "sestina" without a shred of snobbery, and then go on to extol the virtues of the Big Buck Hunter arcade game, without a hint of irony. Joy, suffering, and Pickapeppa Sauce on cream cheese could all be considered in one boozy breath. How many times had I leaned on his barrel chest, scratched first by his bushy red beard, then sandwiched between the arm with the Texas flag and the other with the life-size possum? It was such a relief to surrender to one of his legendary hugs. Without any chance of that physical relief, I hoped his distinct brand of comfort could extend to the phone as well. Though we had not spoken a lot after the rupture, he'd shown his unflagging support from afar, sending me dozens of chapbooks from a variety of poets throughout my recovery. I had never met anyone capable of being so gruff and so kind at the same time. I sensed that his lack of sentimentality might be the only thing that would really counteract the shock of upcoming brain surgery.

Shafer listened to me explain what was going on, with a bartender's patience. He instinctively knew I was seeking his advice, and his grizzled tones were dulcet to me.

Well doll, he said. This can't be easy. But if there's gonna be a showdown between you and some starch-ass surgeon, I'd put all my bets on you. In a mental arm-wrestling contest, you've always been Champeen.

By the end of the conversation, I actually did feel more confident. Shafer had given me the perfect pep talk. I even borrowed some of his irascible language when I faced Dr. Giannotta the next day.

My mother joined me in the exam room. The surgeon's name had sounded Italian to me, but he looked more Irish in person. Freckled, with almost transparent skin, a few years younger than my dad. He shook my hand as he introduced himself, and I started in on my rehearsed cowboy-like resolve, dispensing with all pleasantries.

So? I asked. When do we crack some skulls?

Wh . . . He stumbled. I beg your pardon?

The brain surgery, I said, feeling linguistically leveraged into a position of power. You have to break into my skull, right?

Well, yes, he said, appearing to be reeling slightly from my unexpected introduction. But those aren't the terms we use in the operating room.

Okay, I said, giving him my practiced smile and unflinching gaze. *Craniotomy*, if you prefer.

I was pure cowboy.

Miss Marks, I'm here on the recommendation of my colleague George Teitelbaum, who tells me the coiling you had done six months ago has recanalized.

He told me that too. I am a little confused by that, though. Dr. Teitelbaum saw the scans from Scotland and they appeared to be 100 percent treated.

Dr. Giannotta scoffed. Well, you must've misunderstood. George would never have said that because it's not even possible. With a wide-neck aneurysm like this, there is always a chance of recanalization. The structure is filling with blood again, and the coils that were inserted are now only covering . . . I'd say . . . 75 percent of the aneurysm.

My mother shot me a worried look. Dr. Teitelbaum had already told me that the aneurysm was refilling, but the percentage startled me, too. My brain was only getting a C grade. But I couldn't give in to the fear, and I certainly wasn't going to let this stranger see it.

Fine, I said. If we've got to do this, let's just do it. I was pleased how I was able to utter this statement matter-of-factly, almost nonchalantly.

We haven't even discussed the procedure yet, he protested.

Oh, all right, I allowed. But I have done this sort of thing before.

No, you haven't. Dr. Giannotta's warning was stern. A craniotomy is nothing like a neuroradiological procedure. Not at all.

I'm just saying this isn't my first neurointervention, I hedged, slightly less in control.

You had a primary procedure in Scotland, he interrupted. You need to appreciate that this is a repair job, and an operation over an operation is much more complicated. I'll have to clip over your existing coils and that isn't going to be simple.

He was calling my bluff. He used his freckled, orange fingers to illustrate. The right fist stood for the aneurysm, with two fingers of his left hand against the fist to represent the clamp. He explained that a clip would dam off the aneurysm from the blood flow outside, with the coils remaining inside.

Okay, I said, getting a little queasy from the gory logistics. At least this operation can't be as risky as the one before it.

Why on earth would you think that?

I was momentarily stunned. And then started to feel smaller and smaller with every word I uttered.

Well, uh . . . because . . . well because Scotland was an emergency, I sputtered. Right? And now we have time to plan.

Yes, but Lauren, a procedure like this is pretty rare, he explained. In fact, I'm one of the only surgeons in America who does stuff like this. And I do this every two or three years, at the most. If anything, I'd say this operation is much *more* risky.

And with that single statement, there was no question that I was going to be outmatched in this interaction. The surgeon's self-importance was soaring and mine sinking. The chair beneath me started to feel like a wet sponge. Nothing was quite solid anymore.

But this is something we have to do, I said. I don't have any other options.

Of course you have an option. It's your head. The doctor shrugged, sounding a little disinterested.

This threw me. I didn't want more options in this surgical consult—I wanted *fewer*. I had prepared to be stalwart in the face of a difficult, but inevitable, situation. Instead, I was now being asked to weigh options in a circumstance for which I wasn't at all prepared. And my life depended on making the *right* decision.

You are convinced this is the best course of action? my mother asked him.

We wouldn't be having this conversation if I didn't think that, he said. But you have to fully understand the issues of elective brain surgery. I'm legally obligated to give the risks in a procedure like this. You might end up epileptic, paralyzed, blind. And open brain surgeries are prone to infections—morbidity and mortality rates tend to be high.

Could I lose my language again? I asked. My voice had gotten so tinny and meek.

Oh sure, he said. It's the same location, so that's always a possibility.

My cowboy persona was utterly disarmed at that point, no bullets left in my figurative pistol or spurs on my boots. I simply forced my dry mouth to keep flapping.

When? I asked. When would we do this?

You are going to have to decide that yourself, he said.

I was alarmed. What could he mean? Dr. Giannotta brought his steady hands out again for another example.

As these coils recess, he explained, they give a certain elasticity to the structure itself, which we need because it gives us more room for the operation. Like how you need enough rubber to tie off a water balloon.

As he spoke, I was desperate to catch his eye. I was looking for a comforting sign from him, a friendly twinkle or an empathetic gaze. But there was none to be found.

If we attempt the craniotomy too early, we won't have enough material to do the operation, Dr. Giannotta said. But if we wait too long, you'll have another rupture. And you don't want that, since the chances of survival are extremely low.

Dr. Giannotta seemed completely oblivious to the fact that the information he was conveying was unsettling.

My mother said we'd need a second opinion before we went any further.

Be my guest. I encourage that, but anyone worth their salt will advise you the same way, Dr. Giannotta said. And if you had come through my operating room when the aneurysm ruptured, I would never have put coils in you in the first place.

This comment felt like an insult to me. But the operation in Scotland saved my life! I said, protective of the survival narrative I knew and loved.

Sure it did, Dr. Giannotta said. But they prefer coil embolization over there in Europe, and you shouldn't have a craniotomy if you don't have a very experienced surgeon available, that's for sure. But if you had been here in the US, I would've clipped that aneurysm then and there, and you wouldn't have any of these complications now. Anything we are going to do from this point on is going to be . . . tricky.

Though the aneurysm in my brain was holding, this was when the dam of terror in me finally broke. And with that, all the confidence I had been building up in my journal started to slip away too.

-over-riding narrative competing narrative
Is this a recovery story?

almost no sleep. fear. true fear.

the situation has not changed since yesterday. the medical situation. but the conversation with the neurosurgeon risky. only does it once every 2 or 3 years. problem of my agency. asked me to re-evaluate the surgery. Do I have any choice? Why is he giving me choices?

A Tale of Two Aneurysms. I for me, the story of the coiled aneurysm is miraculous. It is illuminating. It is enlightening. But Dr. Giaattano?

changes the story of the aneursym, No, it is not getting better. No, it is not
going to get better. He troubles my experience, he troubles my center.

The need for a second surgery was eroding the sense of meaning I had
acquired after the rupture. It was that simple and that profound.

Until my appointment with Dr. Giannotta, I had felt like I had been
part of a story that made sense. This story was about a young woman who
had loved words and then her words had been taken away from her. She
worked hard to return what was lost, and in the meanwhile, she was able
to encounter her language in a wholly different way. She was writing her
way back to fluency.

There was symmetry in that story, with lessons to learn, and I could
easily situate myself inside of it. A dramatic event had taken place and it
had changed the course of my life. But I had also been in the right place,
at the right time, and I had come to believe that I was the right person as
well. I hadn't minded the trials of my recovery because they had ultimately
bolstered my sense of purpose and certainty. My faulty brain was repairing
itself, making a more sophisticated version of what it used to be. I was more
curious, more confident, and more comfortable than I ever had been before.

But once I found out that there was a dramatic failing in the very part
of my brain I had treated with such reverence, what I had experienced
as fate suddenly seemed nothing more than delusion. I didn't feel part of
some magnificent sense of order, but instead like an insignificant person
whose life events were entirely random. The apparent absurdity of writing
my way through this linguistic recovery only highlighted this sudden sense
of worthlessness. What recovery? Dr. Giannotta himself had said that I
might not be able to use language again after I woke up from the surgery.
If I woke up at all. The journal entries wouldn't lead up to anything else;
whatever ideas started in there would most likely remain unfinished. There
was no Quiet to find comfort in.

My stable sleep schedule turned erratic and then became nonexistent.
If I somehow managed to doze off watching late-night TV, I'd wake up

abruptly, my heart pounding. I'd swallow over-the-counter sleeping pills to make my eyes close. The words the surgeon had used to describe the upcoming procedure haunted me. *Risky,* he had said. *Tricky.* The terms sounded like names of rodeo ponies. Something whimsical, even playful. The operation was anything but.

I'd always thought of the second aneurysm as more dangerous than the first. The latter had, in so many ways, made me who I was. But now, to hear that it was threatening my current life? And everything I'd built up over the past several months? It was a betrayal of the highest order.

Both of my parents came to the second surgical consult at the University of California, Los Angeles.

We sat anxiously in the exam room and after thirty minutes heard a soft double knock on the door. We all stiffened. When the door actually opened, we were surprised to see a young administrator in khakis. He popped his head in, without stepping foot into the room. Sorry for the wait, he said. The doctor will be with you soon.

In the course of the next hour, we all changed positions: standing, stalking, pacing. Then there was the same double knock, and the same lower functionary giving us the same misguided update. Sorry for the wait, he repeated. The doctor will be with you soon.

"Waiting" became a pretty abstract concept after two and a half hours.

When the all-too-anticipated rap came again, my father opened the door himself, which surprised the administrator. Let me guess, Dad said, with no small amount of sarcasm. The doctor will be here soon?

That's right, the man said, as he threaded his thumb through one of his belt loops. Soon.

Waiting for Godot in here, Dad muttered after he left. Paging Dr. Godot . . .

Cabin fever was setting in. I started to snoop through the doctor's cupboards and drawers, and I grabbed a disposable plastic cone meant for ear and nose examinations. I flipped it around, and put it on one of my eyes, like a plastic monocle. I offered my parents invisible tea from the surgical sink, and we all giggled like we were on laughing gas. I was so grateful for them in that moment. Not just for being with me, but for indulging this frivolity. It gave me a tiny distraction before facing some unknowable future. I felt lucky to be inside a family unwilling to surrender their moments of joy, however small or fleeting.

I don't remember what we were doing when the surgeon actually arrived, but he was four and a half hours late. And he didn't feel compelled to give us any explanation for his delay. At that point, I'd already been introduced to the brusque manner and distracted attitude of a neurosurgeon. Though Dr. Martin's demeanor was as similarly unsociable as Dr. Giannotta's, I was starting to think he was just playing to type. Martin popped my scans into a drive and displayed them on a large screen.

What do you think? I asked him.

Well, there is no question that you need an operation soon, he answered. Speak to the secretary up front and she'll put you on my calendar. He stood up, as if ready to leave.

Hold up for a second, my dad said. We still have a couple of questions. Lauren is still deciding where she wants to do the surgery. You are our second opinion.

Oh really? The surgeon's keen eyes narrowed. Who else are you considering? Because this is a very delicate procedure, you know. Not everybody does this.

She's been speaking to Dr. Giannotta, my mother answered. At USC.

Hmpf. The surgeon exhaled his disapproval through his nose, a kind of bull-snort. Yeah. Dr. Giannotta is probably the only other guy who could do this.

Do you think it should happen soon? my father asked.

I'd expect so, the surgeon said. Can't say exactly when. But waiting too long . . . well, you just can't wait too long.

23

A few days after my second surgery consult, I got a pleasant surprise when my friend Rachel came to LA for a visit. Her husband was in San Francisco at the time, so it was an easy journey down. Like many of my friends, Rachel and I met as performers at NYU, and we were even in a couple of plays together. But Rachel had been an actor's actor back in school, tending to get cast in some of the bigger productions, on the larger stages. And after graduation, when she discovered she was no longer being cast in the roles she wanted, she started writing plays herself, creating the kind of characters she liked and worlds she wanted to inhabit. With a talent for re-invention, she soon shifted her entire focus to writing. Now she had written a memoir, and had meetings in LA to prepare for her first book tour. She intuited that things might be a little tense in my household, so she had decided to stay with one of her pals in Venice Beach. But she still wanted to see me. And since I had recently been granted full freeway privileges, I offered to meet her by the ocean.

I was sitting on the patio at a beachfront café when Rachel was dropped off. It was the first time we'd seen each other since my post-surgical stop in New York. When she spotted me, she beelined for the table, but a blonde in a bikini top and a group of half-nude teenagers toting boogie boards almost knocked her over. When Rachel finally arrived at the table, she was flustered, and readjusted the neckline of her faded Morrissey T-shirt.

Is it a crime to be a brunette in this town or something? she asked. With all these sun-kissed, tight-bunned Aryans scampering about, you and I must look like Morticia Adams.

It was an off-the-cuff comment, but invoking this corpse-like character spurred a bleak thought in me: this could be my very last conversation with Rachel. I couldn't help but start to imagine the sort of things I'd have to say to her, and everyone, if I was never going to speak to them again. I would tell my brother to take care of our parents and himself. I would tell my parents that I had taken chances, followed whims, that I had loved and been loved, and they should never imagine my life as unlived. And Jonah. I'd have to say something to Jonah.

I knew it was morbid, but all the internal language that filtered through my now-working inner voice was fixated on the catastrophic. I forced my attention back to Rachel and the sea breeze. She was telling me that she had just finished editing the memoir she wrote, and that there was a surprise for me inside it.

You are in my memoir, you know, and I was just thinking that while you are recuperating from surgery, you can read about yourself in a book! That's a little glamorous, right? Just like a movie star.

If I can still read, I said.

Rachel's alarm shot through her face, and her lips went as blue as her eyes.

Oh, honey, she said, trying to cover up her concern. Don't say that. Of course you'll still be able to read.

Rachel's presence was a comfort, but we were living in two different worlds. I was proud of her and her recent accomplishments—it was her first book, after all, and writing it had been no easy feat—but I couldn't help but be nervous about the whole thing. She had this complete, intact version of me in her pages, something I hardly had access to myself. From what I could understand, the memoir focused on the time before

the aneurysm had ruptured and featured many of the intoxicated mis-
adventures of our early twenties. I feared her character of me was going
to outlive the real me, and I might not ever be able to put forth my own
alternative.

She reached across the table and grabbed for my hand. Hospital or no
hospital, I'm going to come visit you after the surgery, she promised. I'm
coming back to LA very soon. Okay? I'm always here for you, lovey.

After a long lunch, Rachel's friend came back to pick her up. We said
good-bye, but I decided to linger on the beach a bit longer. I had scheduled
a phone call with an old classmate from NYU who had also undergone
a craniotomy a couple of years earlier. She had been my scene partner in
some of our acting classes, and we had celebrated our first Thanksgiving
in New York together, eventually becoming very close friends. But she had
developed a very rare neurological condition our sophomore year, which
was detected early and operated on successfully. At the time, it was the talk
of the whole theater department. She recovered and returned to school as
if nothing had happened. Her case was very different from my own, but I
needed a sounding board, someone who at least could imagine and understand what I might be going through.

I pulled out my cell phone and dialed. The first thing I did when she
answered was apologize. Life after school had pulled us in different directions, and we had hardly touched base since then. I felt bad that I'd been
so remiss in keeping in contact, and that this was going to be our first
conversation in a while.

No sweat, she said. Nothing brings people together like neurosurgery.

I guess that's true. I laughed. It is pretty hard to talk about the details
of this with most people.

Oh yeah, she said. I had no filter about that for a while myself. But I
found out the hard way that not a lot of people want to chat about bone-
saws over cocktails and canapés. Still, I am not squeamish at all, so just ask
anything you want to ask.

I guess I want to know how, I began. How . . . How did you prepare
yourself to do this?

I hoped she'd have the kind of wisdom of experience that everyone else lacked.

Let's see, she said, casting her memory several years back. Honestly, I think all I did was buy a pair of rollerblades and some new pajamas. Nice things that I could wake up to in the hospital.

What do you mean? I asked. Was that all you did?

Basically yeah, she said. Beforehand, I just pretended the whole thing wasn't happening.

It didn't seem possible. This was the very definition of a life-changing event, and my pal was telling me that her only preparation for it was some light retail therapy.

This surgery threatened your life and your livelihood, I said. You aren't actually suggesting that you found a way to *ignore* it. . . .

That's exactly what I'm saying, Lauren. We all do this sort of thing in our own way. For me? I discovered that De-Nile ain't just a river in Egypt.

Stunned by her comment, I found even the suggestion of this kind of approach completely appalling. Whatever I was facing, I didn't think I was capable of ignoring it, even if I tried. The only way out was through.

24

In the weeks leading up to the surgery, Jonah and I had started to bicker, and the main point of contention was logistics. He couldn't book his ticket to LA until I had sorted out the details of the operation. But I hadn't decided who would do the surgery, let alone where or when.

The end of the month, I told him. Or early April. Maybe you should carve out a couple of weeks, with some flexible dates for your arrival and departure.

Lauren, I cannot get a ticket like that, Jonah said. I've got to make a living out here. Not trying to upset you, but it feels a little like you're being intentionally evasive. . . .

He wasn't exactly wrong. But there was a reason for me to be cagey, and I was irritated that Jonah didn't sense it. I simply didn't want to discuss this topic more. There was a lot of subtext that I needed Jonah to read into without me explaining. "A couple of weeks" could allow for a prolonged coma. "Flexible" could even include a funeral. It is safe to say that my fears had become overly fatalistic, but I refused to be any more linguistically clear because airing those fears in the world, in that way, would only give them more power over me.

I know this is difficult for you, Lauren. But it is kind of like you don't even want me there, he continued.

This is not what this is about! I said, surprised by the exasperation in my voice. I knew it wasn't a simple trip for Jonah. But the fact was I would prefer him not to come if he was going to make things harder instead of easier.

If this is too complicated, Jo, I promise I won't blame you if you can't be here.

And there you go again, he said. I really want to be at your side, Lauren. I really do. You keep cutting me off at the pass, though, so I guess I have to ask: Why wouldn't you want me there?

It was so hard to convey what it was like for me at this moment to Jonah. I felt so off-balance, even a small gust of wind, from any direction, could shatter me into pieces. I did want Jonah to come to California, but I couldn't let him be the linchpin either—because I had to be fine even if he didn't come, too.

Though my friend who had also gone through a craniotomy extolled the virtues of denial, I found this forced forgetfulness impossible. I desperately wanted to seek out the comforting order of the Quiet. But I wasn't even sure what that was anymore. Delusion? Invention? I wasn't even sure if I should want to want the Quiet. Jonah became a convenient scapegoat for my helplessness. After yet another conversation had gone wrong, he tried to apologize via text, but I furiously scribbled my frustration about him in my journal, and tried to find the words I should have told him when I could.

"I'm sorry i was short with you. I'll try to call later."
a text from Jonah

He was short. In a conversation about travel plans to L.A. I said he could book a ticket with putting it on hold, instead of pay for it up front. This is because I haven't decide on the date of the surgery, because I haven't decide my surgeon. I he said something about "not able to be to flexible" and a glib "I have to make a living over here." His curt comment leave me hurt and angry. I've told he doesn't need to go come.

But I need to say is plainly I will not bedgrudge if you do or you don't.
But if you are going to be here, you must support me. Visualizing the punk
rock haircut, the long bandaged scar. Visualizing the room in the hospital
and the view outside. Visualize an extremely successful surgery. Walking,
unsteadily, down halls ~~of the~~ From the I.C.U. Visualizing me parents~~Tell~~
Tell me if I should in corporate in the landscape.

The journal didn't much help with my visualizing exercise—all I
wanted to do was create an image of myself waking up from surgery. And
the more detailed the better. But when Jonah and I were arguing, I kept
inserting and removing him from this image, which frustrated me to no
end. Whatever, I thought. Fuck. This.

25

In many ways, Dr. Russin had become the axle of my medical wheel in Los Angeles. She was the first person to be on my "team," before the neuro-radiologist, neurosurgeon, neuropsychologist, or even Justine signed on to the case. My surgical deliberations had been hugely counterproductive thus far, as I continued like a windup toy, hitting the same wall over and over, maddened by the amount of information I could so easily find online but not so easily interpret. It seemed you needed to study brain science before you could actually select a brain surgeon. I walked outside into my mother's rose garden in full bloom and called Dr. Russin.

I had my second opinion, I told her. At UCLA.

And?

Still can't decide.

Listen, Lauren, she said. The surgery is a given. And these are both very reputable surgeons, so you just have to choose between them.

I just don't know what I am supposed to do.

And I really didn't. This is what I knew about my two potential neurosurgeons: They were both placed at high-profile universities. They were both the chairmen of their respective programs. They had world-class reputations. And I had to trust one of them with my life. The stakes couldn't be any higher. Their credentials were undeniable, but the problem was that I didn't especially like either of them.

USC or UCLA. USC or UCLA. I waffled back and forth. USC and UCLA had a famous rivalry, known since birth by kids who grew up in Los Angeles, where allegiances were declared through shirts and bumper stickers. On game days, flags would be unfurled in neighbors' yards. Even children in elementary school were expected to choose sides. I didn't care about sports at all and I had no fixed allegiance, but since my father had pursued a master's in theater at UCLA, it was my default school when pressed for playground fealty. Could I actually let a university rivalry inform my choice of a neurosurgeon? Irrationally, I caught myself doing exactly that. I was even weighing the values of the schools' mascots against each other. Bruin versus Trojan: cheery teddy bear versus Roman soldier. At least a Trojan had experience with sharp instruments, and had opposable thumbs. That was a plus.

I hoped Dr. Russin could be more practical.

The doctors won't even look me in the eye! I complained. How am I supposed to trust my life to someone who won't even meet my gaze?

That's hard, I know. But you don't choose your surgeon because of his bedside manner, she said. You choose him for his hands.

What would *you* do?

Dr. Russin sighed. Well, I have a cousin out in Nevada. She had a neurosurgery botched out there, and I brought her to LA because it was clear she needed another operation. Lots of people vouch for the excellence of the UCLA team. But when it came down to my own family member, I went with USC and sent her off to Giannotta. Afterward, I saw the video of his surgery. He's ambidextrous, just as good with his left wrist as his right. A pure artist.

Finally, I was getting information that seemed relevant to me.

And, she added, Dr. Giannotta doesn't mess around with drugs or booze. I am certainly not saying that Martin doesn't either, I just don't know him that well. Surgeons are just people, like all of us. You've got to consider all the factors. And I know Dr. Giannotta better.

I started to hyperventilate. Jesus—it never occurred to me before then—but there were neurosurgeons who might come into the operating theater drunk? Or high? In addition to investigating their professional credentials, should I be asking about their personal lives too? Did anyone have a sick parent—or a wife who was leaving him for a younger man? It was too much to take in. If I were a windup toy, this was a ham-fisted turn of my key.

It was the first time I had allowed myself to cry since I found out about the craniotomy, and I started to weep. I didn't want to be too emotional in front of my family because it might bring out their own hysterics. But the confusion, the distress—it all became salt water. My heaves made the phone slick with my tears.

Dr. Russin softened her voice. It's okay to cry, she said. If it were me, I might be crying too.

This made me cry even more.

But by the end of the call, I had finally made my decision.

It had been hard to explain to Krass why I wanted to go to the Paris catacombs in the first place, especially since he had been initially reluctant. It seemed to me that it was as big a draw as any other tourist site there. So much of Parisian existence celebrated life, but it was one of the few major cities that preserved such a profound reminder of death, too. Also, there was something I had always loved about transitional spaces, from buildings in construction to long-abandoned ruins. Their history and potential was intoxicating. After some convincing, Krass begrudgingly decided to join me.

When we arrived at the red brick entrance, we descended the winding stone staircases into the dimly lit underground. Krass translated the plaque before us, which warned us not to take, or touch, anything.

Six million dead Parisians were housed in the catacombs, resting three stories below the city. The first items we saw were some large bones, specimens tucked away in dim enclaves. We had to peer through bars to observe them. But after that, there was a major transformation of space. There was a huge volume of bones that were no longer kept in separate rooms; they were just stacked. There were skulls everywhere, skulls without bodies attached, ceiling-to-floor skulls. They were piled on top of each other, creating the very walls of the tunnel, sometimes assembled in geometric shapes and aesthetically constructed rows like mandalas of human parts.

I slowed down to a reverent pace. I started to crouch every few yards to imagine flesh on the skeletal remains, reminding myself these were people, not wallpaper. This man, I imagined, was a merchant who died from influenza and was survived by his plump wife with a goiter. This was a girl who had been skipping by the Seine in a rainstorm and had tumbled unnoticed under the water, her body not found for weeks. How many people died together, in war or fire or plague? I was especially drawn to a skull on the floor with a hole inside of it, slightly larger than a kernel of corn. It was a smallish specimen. I decided it was a woman, and there was no reason to concoct the cause of her death—the desiccated bullet wound an inch above her right eye socket was explanation enough. With no docent hovering nearby, I slipped my pinky finger into the skull. I didn't lift it from its place, but could feel its ridged and dear weight, like a ring on my finger.

Nothing about this touch felt like a trespass. But for a few short seconds, the woman and I were as closely linked as any human beings could be. Her life and death were suddenly part of me, too, and with such an allegiance between us, contemplating my own eventual death didn't seem so horrible.

Krass was no longer beside me, but I knew there was no chance of us losing each other. In spite of the labyrinthine turns of the sepulcher, there was only one way out, if you were getting out. When I finally climbed the winding stone stairs, I found him in the gift shop. He looked pale as he fiddled with the music boxes.

We sat down for a drink at the nearest bar where he proclaimed that he would never take that trip again. Not for all the oolong in China, he swore.

From his red barstool, I could tell he was waiting for a tacit agreement from me. When I didn't offer it, he prodded. Oh, come on, Lauren, he said. You can't just tell me that you felt absolutely *fine* in that place.

But I had been.

Sometimes I wonder if the peaceful sensations I had experienced were somehow related to the pressure building so quietly in my brain. Physiologically, my life was in imminent danger when I was in Paris, I just was not consciously aware of it yet. I had been rummaging inside of a woman's skull and in a couple of weeks, others would be rummaging through mine. But how utterly strange to think of it like that. Part of me wants to believe I was preparing myself for things to come, and the reason I felt surprisingly comfortable in the catacombs was a pre-recognition, or some kind of prescience.

Still, I know that hindsight can be sneaky that way. Every event that starts as random and disconnected is later drawn to have direct links in the minds of those recalling it.

The magnitude of the tomb did stir something in me, but what was it exactly?

And I wanted Krass to understand. I felt solemn, I said. Sort of . . . safe.

26

The evening after my neurosurgical discussion with Dr. Russin, I slept soundly. Deciding on USC and the date of the procedure had helped, too, and the nightmares that had been plaguing me since my consult with Dr. Giannotta relented a bit. Gratefully refreshed the next morning, I told my parents that I'd join them on their morning walk, as soon as I had jotted down the details of the dream I'd had the night before:

Dream

Mom buys a new house, but doesn't have the money do-t it. It could be an huge investment but with rixks. I wonder over the rooms, inspecting the newness—built up to the qualifications.

I have to remove my books from my treehouse. All paperbacks. Illustration with caption—two kids on the tricicylues talking about the Odyssey and (Illid?). I want to ge with a my books out of the treehouse in one trip. walking up the slide.

an older mustaschioed man tries to help me but he can't climb the slide. I
catch a foot into a step, and the other leg in perpindicular fashion, a ferry
the books this way. upside down. right side up. upside down. right side up.

The dream didn't bring up a lot of reactions in me. In fact, it was somewhat straightforward, symbolically. Treehouse = head. Book = knowledge.
The risks of moving to a new house = brain surgery. When I finished writing
it all down, I joined my parents outside. But today we were also picking up
our friend's dog, so our route changed slightly. On the way down the street,
we passed a sun-bleached red Toyota, parked not far from our own driveway.
From behind the car, I could see the driver's head slightly bowed. Sleeping?
Listening to the radio? A red book was on the dashboard, bouncing pink
light against the windshield. Nothing seemed to be out of the ordinary or
out of place, really. And then I saw his mustache. That changed everything.

That guy, I told my parents. That guy was in my dream last night.

He looks like someone from your dream, my mom said. Huh. That's
weird.

I faced the car again. No, I told her. It doesn't *look* like that guy—it *is*
that guy.

Are you really positive? she asked, intrigued.

Hate to burst anybody's bubble here, my father interrupted, but Lauren isn't positive because she can't be positive about something impossible.
This is just one of the many ways the mind can be suggestible.

Though these people were our neighbors, I hadn't met them before.
My parents didn't know them well either, but they explained to me that this
group had an early-morning prayer breakfast once a month. My parents
had always found them to be kind and cordial, but that was basically the
extent of what they knew.

The dog down the road was eagerly awaiting our arrival, and I helped
my parents put him on a leash. When we passed the red car again five minutes later, the man was getting out of it. I rushed over to meet him.

Hi, I said, extending my hand. How are you?

Oh! The man was surprised, but shook my hand immediately. He then searched my face for any sign of recognition. I am . . . quite . . . well, thanks. And you?

My parents apologized for my abrupt introduction and introduced themselves as well.

My folks think I'm crazy, I said hesitantly. And maybe you'll think I'm crazy, too. But you were in my dream last night.

To my great relief, he wasn't put off by the comment. Instead, it seemed to tickle him. His laugh was warm and welcoming. I guess I should be honored! he said. He introduced himself as Reverend Meyers, and I asked him about the morning meeting. Was it some sort of prayer group, like my parents said?

Not exactly, he said. Wednesdays are oatmeal days. He explained that the group was nondenominational and consisted mainly of peace and justice workers, some of whom worked in religious groups, others in more secular environments. But they were all people of faith.

You are welcome to join us any time you'd like.

I looked to my folks and the panting dog and made the split-second decision to give up on the walk and join this stranger's gathering. It was clear that Reverend Meyers didn't expect me to join them right away. His kind expression was infused with an equal mix of confusion and amusement.

My mother leaped in to save me any potential embarrassment. Unless of course you'd rather just have your regular meeting without distractions, she said.

Not at all, the man said. Your daughter should definitely come in. The more the merrier!

I can't say what moved me to be so forward, but my mind had been mired in the sludge for weeks, and the excitement of being exposed to something a bit uncanny was intriguing. Inside the house, everyone made room for me at the table. A group member grabbed a chair for me, another gave me a bowl and a spoon, and someone else poured my orange juice. Most of them were around my grandma's age and several conversations were already underway. A woman in dangly earrings was talking about the housing crisis in Los Angeles and how she was letting a homeless man stay with her until he was placed in a proper care facility. A couple at the head of the table—my neighbors, I later discovered—were discussing the decades of strife after the CIA-driven coup in Guatemala. A bald man detailed his upcoming trip to the Palestinian territories, and the people around him were debating whether Israeli actions in the area amounted to prosecutable war crimes. The subject matter made it all sound more like a political science class than a prayer meeting.

A huge pot of pecan oatmeal was resting on the table, and Reverend Meyers offered some to me. I thanked him but told him I was allergic. He wasted no time grabbing a smaller pot from inside the kitchen.

You are in luck, he said. Sister Pat doesn't take nuts either, so we've got our bases covered here. He gave me a ladle full of porridge.

He nodded to the woman beside me, her grey hair in a boyish cut. After our bowls were filled, I tried to engage the nun in conversation, asking how everyone in the group knew each other.

Oh, us? We're just a ragtag group of troublemakers, she said, giving me a wizened wink. Let's see, some people met at divinity school at Harvard, some during their missionary work in Central America, and others were picked up at human rights protests, or events like that.

But you are a Catholic nun, aren't you? I asked.

Until I hear otherwise! Her throaty, joyful voice resounded in the room. There are usually a couple of Catholic nuns at this gathering, she explained. But there are also Presbyterians, Lutherans, Anglicans. We don't have any priests in attendance, though we've got several retired pastors.

When the group got around to asking me questions, I felt strangely comfortable telling my story, from the surgery in Scotland to the upcoming operation. Even in my very short time in this room, I had already heard stories from people who had survived kidnappings, rocket launches, and bomb blasts. I only felt easy sharing my personal experiences when I could trust that it wouldn't make me the center of attention or a source of pity. My story was hardly the most interesting or the most perilous. Everyone listened attentively, responded graciously, and then they all moved on to the other items of the day. It couldn't have gone any better.

It was an informal affair, without Bible verses or sermons. Instead, they discussed urgent community concerns, some local, some global, and the members decided among themselves what resources could be committed to what causes. As the conversations wound down, and the bowls were returned to the kitchen, I leaned over to Sister Pat again.

I didn't know what it was about her that made her easy to talk to. Perhaps it was her weathered look that reminded me that she had endured all manner of things already, a face that looked like it had a talent for keeping confidences. Also, I had let a dream guide me into this space, so it seemed important that I make the best of my time in here. I told the nun that since the paperwork at the angiogram required me to state my faith, I'd started thinking about religion again.

That's understandable, dear, she said. Before major life changes, a lot of people feel compelled to make peace with their faith.

Make peace. The phrase struck me as interesting. Faith is fragmented, with moments of illumination and moments of murk. It could be like a cracked mirror—one could see oneself in it, but only in shards. I couldn't imagine anyone making *peace* with their faith, only *pieces.*

My mother had been a liberal Catholic my whole life, my father an agnostic, and although I was a somewhat contrary teenager, I loved studying religions. I understood how the dogma, shame, and violence so often associated with religion put many people off. But what intrigued me most was mysticism, specifically the idea of transcendence. Every major religion in the world contains literature about the breaking down of barriers between the self and something larger, and that belief is anti-dogmatic at its very core. So much of religion is about laying down rules of obedience, prescribing the acceptable ways of worship, and outlining the relationship between creator and creation. But in a moment of transcendence, such distinctions dissolve. During a *unio mystica*, it is impossible to know the difference between self and other, or man and God. To be clear, becoming "one with God" actually borders on heresy in monotheistic traditions because it jeopardizes the very idea of God's unique oneness. Yet, most of these same religions have saints who reported transcendent experiences and went on to be revered as holy people, as opposed to heretics. I just loved that. That meant their experience both confirmed and contradicted some of the most sacred tenants of their belief systems. God was God, and humans were humans, except when they weren't. Still, using language to describe transcendence made for a fraught translation; too much was lost between the finite and the infinite.

I hadn't put my neurological condition into this specific religious context before, but thinking about transcendence again, there were many similarities. It did alter my consciousness, changing my sense of self and my sense of the world. And it certainly showed me the limits of language inside something much more vast.

As much as I was indulging in a theological thought pattern again, it didn't mean I wasn't afraid of my upcoming surgery. I was petrified.

So I marshaled a question I had been too nervous to ask the nun initially. Considering the risks at hand, Sister, I said, do you think I should go to confession before the surgery?

Well, she said. It depends on what you want from a confession.

I thought this was a stunning thing for a nun to say. She didn't say: That is your role as a Catholic or: You should if you fear for your immortal soul, but what *I would want* from a confession. I was well aware that I had participated in plenty of activities that the Catholic Church would deem necessary to confess, but I was also sure the church and I defined "sin" differently. I told Sister Pat that I had shortcomings, plenty of them. But nothing burdened my conscience. I honestly felt I had nothing to confess.

Sounds like you answered your own question, she said as she patted my back with a strong, wide palm. There is no hard and fast rule about absolution. I can easily get you in contact with a good priest, if you'd like, even if you just want to talk. But remember you've landed in the clutch of some radicals, and at this very table, there are nuns who have given communion to non-Catholics. Not naming names, of course! Just take comfort that you are surrounded by people who don't always color within the lines.

Reverend Meyers, the man with the mustache who brought me into this group, emerged from my neighbors' kitchen, a dishtowel slung over his shoulder.

Thanks for letting me come, I said. Sorry if I was weird.

Nonsense. The pastor dried his hands. We loved having you and we hope you'll come back. Anytime.

As I returned to my own driveway, I had a lot to think about—it wasn't like everything had fallen completely into place. But what was thrilling, though, was that I felt I *could* think again.

No one in the group had tried to dispense tired bromides to me like, "It's all part of God's grand plan." I probably would've responded very poorly if they had. From imagining my last words, to obsessive and unproductive research about possible complications of the procedure, my inner and outer language had kept me on a hamster wheel of anxiety. But I knew that calculating my own worst case scenarios wouldn't keep them from happening. And having no faith in myself, no faith in the Quiet, no faith in anything, had only crippled my sense of purpose and meaning. I realized that the most radical thought I could think was this: that everything was exactly as it should be.

And regardless of the outcome of the procedure, at this point fighting or fixating couldn't serve me as much as trusting. All I could do now was submit.

27

F̶The neurosurgeon tells me that I might have to return to speech therapy.
Bj says that seems unfair, "d̶Does it trouble you." That fear? <u>Minor, in</u>
<u>*compare to f̶e the fear of all fears*</u>*. What about it? If I have to do it?*
My memories tell me that I loved the experiences through the language
returning, discovering. I say "maybe that it might be like falling in love
again."

T̶h̶e̶ ̶s̶e̶c̶o̶n̶d̶ I contemplate a possible second time. There is thrill, there
is attraction, there is excitement of unknown. But the question of
singularity. The first time everything feels stuffed with magic and fate,
destination. The second time, the mystery is still excitable, but knows that
us is not once in a lifetime, It is r̶e̶p̶e̶a̶t̶a̶b̶l̶e̶ groungeable outlineable. And
yet, we do. We fall again, and grateful the opportunity to do so.

Though I was slowly coming around to accepting my upcoming surgery,
considering the idea that I might have to return to speech therapy after
the fact presented more complicated feelings. As much as I had wanted
to stay in speech therapy a month ago, starting all over from scratch was

a different thing entirely. I had done this work already. Having relearned language after the rupture felt meaningful, even triumphant. But imagining that I might have to do it all again, and so soon after my graduation, felt Sisyphean. It was enough to keep me spinning. So when a moment of panic about the surgery arose, I would consciously try to adjust my internal reaction to keep it from exaggerating itself. This was a technique I called *duck thinking* because of something I had been exposed to a few months earlier.

One rainy day, late in the afternoon, I had noticed a black van parked right in front of my parents' house. I hadn't seen it arrive, but even in the pouring rain I could see that the driver was still inside. I sat at the desk in my red bedroom, alone in the house, watching the silhouette of the man doing God only knew what.

The van drove away at some point, and it was still raining when I fell asleep. But late in the night, a jarring bump from outside woke me up. I heard a rubbery slosh, like something heavy dragging in the driveway. My imagination sprang into action. Was that the sound a human body would make if it were in a trash bag being hauled through puddles?

My bed was situated between two windows that faced the driveway—a clear enough view to the street, even in the mist. All I needed to do was to get out of bed and raise the shades, but a paralysis kept me exactly where I was. I wanted to go to the window, but I was too afraid of what I might find.

Then, I had an idea. If my mind had suggested a particularly negative scenario, it should be able to imagine an equally positive one, a counterbalance that would relax me. A replacement.

I started to concoct an alternate story that was completely devoid of menace. I told myself that in the high winds a Little Tikes play set had blown in from a neighbor's yard. The plastic slide accounted for the rubbery aspect. There were bodies in this scenario, too, but they were not people, and they were certainly not dead. They were a family of ducks, and they had co-opted the child's toy as their own. The dragging sound I had heard transformed into a slipping one. The mother duck was climbing the short, blue ladder to arrive at the orange slide. She was instructing her ducklings how to take the chute, webbed feet up.

This elaborate storytelling exercise changed everything. I was emboldened enough to leave the bed. When I arrived at the window, I was unafraid, and was able to discover that the driveway was empty.

I had forgotten about the ducks for a while, and certainly hadn't been able to use the technique right after the craniotomy consults. But now, I was happy to invite them back into my life.

It didn't have to be ducks, of course, but I found them pretty reliable as a touchstone. So whenever I got overwhelmed, I guided my mind to ducks. Cartoon ducks, usually. They wore scuba gear or tutus, they played brass instruments, they smoked cigars, and they were incredibly gassy. Words weren't welcome in these animated sequences, just bright, silly images. This helped reverse the anxiety cycle for a little while. After those shorts played out in my brain, I still needed to face the issues at hand, but I could do so with a much more relaxed mind.

One of my biggest anxieties was that Dr. Giannotta had warned I might lose my language again. But with a calmer mind, I was able to investigate what made this threat so scary.

Would I be able to commit to my language practice again? Probably. Would I resent everything I had come to enjoy about my former lessons? Possibly, but it seemed unlikely. Would I come to hate language itself for dragging me through its elaborate obstacle course another time? Definitely not. I might have to return to where I came from, but was that so bad? It hadn't been the worst place to land.

I thought it might be a little like falling in love again.

Your first love feels everlasting, until it's over. The end of it is shocking because the experience had felt so pure and incorruptible. The second time is different. The concept of permanency is porous because even as you have this magnificent sensation and the variety of sub-sensations that stem from it, you know it all can change. Still, despite the knowledge that this love might end, you let it in again. Pain is possible, you know that now, but you still want to feel the exhilaration and the tenderness regardless. Hope re-emerges in you. Perhaps you tend to this love differently and find new ways of relishing it. You learn by doing, and as long as you keep learning, you pick up different things the second time.

But you still fall. And it's still love. And nothing will ever be better than that.

28

It was only after I had finalized my surgical plans in mid-March that I remembered Materson's trip. He had been visiting Laura and BJ in New York, but I hadn't consulted with him about the dates I'd selected for my surgery. And I realized that his vacation in LA would directly correspond with my operation, which concerned me. I wanted to cultivate a certain amount of solemnity in my immediate area. But my brother was coming, Jonah was coming—making it already a full house—and now with Materson, too, there was a variety of personalities and temperaments that I feared might clash. I just didn't want too many variables.

Depending on the outcome of the procedure, it could be an awkward period to be a houseguest, so before Materson bought a plane ticket to California, I gently mentioned to him that it might be best if he considered changing his plans a bit.

Why? he innocently asked me. Is the operation super serious?

His comment struck me as endearing because, after all, he knew exactly what serious could mean in this context. He had already observed it firsthand. It was an enjoyable mental exercise, trying to imagine myself from Materson's perspective. When I observed my own life in its entirety, the events of these brain surgeries couldn't be any more dramatic. But Materson had hardly known me "before." These operations were simply part of the character he understood me as. Lauren Marks: brown hair, hazel eyes, red lipstick, prone to neurosurgeries. It didn't faze him at all. Materson wanted to keep his trip as planned, so I stopped trying to dissuade him.

When I picked him up from the Burbank airport a couple of weeks later, he was in a weathered sweatshirt and a beanie, looking floppy as a Muppet. He exuded this relaxed, lively energy, which made me glad I hadn't kept him away. My pleasure only increased when Jonah flew in the next day. As soon as I had fixed all of the elements of my procedure in place, he and I had gotten back into sync. Before these visitors arrived, I had assumed that I'd need some monastic quiet, and razor-sharp focus, to prepare myself for the upcoming surgery, but the company was also a welcome distraction. The boys had met briefly in Scotland, so they reconnected with ease, and once my brother arrived from Monterey, he and Materson also became fast friends. Everyone in the house adapted to the best ways to cohabitate.

One afternoon, Materson came across me in the kitchen while I prepared to confront my surgical packet. I sighed at the weight of it.

You're not getting nervous about the brain surgery, are you? Materson asked. Because you are an old pro!

Though Dr. Giannotta had told me this surgery was as dangerous—or more dangerous—than the first one, it seemed to me that most of the people around me were not experiencing the same uncertainty this time around. As they understood it, my second operation was minor in comparison to the first one since at least this time we were all prepared. In a much more acute way, I realized that I had been completely spared of the terror my loved ones had suffered while I was in Scotland. When I considered the second surgery, my natural fear would creep in sometimes, but it also felt appropriate that I go through this myself. It seemed only fair that it was my turn being scared. My turn to doubt.

The weeks before the surgery became partially filled by presidential primaries in my household, our TVs blaring information about potential candidates in both parties, all of us taken by the historic overtones of this race. My mother, grandmother, and I all often watched together, and although I was casting my lot with Obama and they were Clinton supporters, we all respected both candidates. But after one debate, when it was becoming clear that Hillary Clinton was losing ground and was not going to be nominated as the candidate for this election, my mother became decidedly less diplomatic in her opinions about this primary process. She made a remark on the blatant misogyny Clinton had been subjected to throughout and as my mom's face reddened, she announced that she needed to go outside for some air. I proposed joining her for a walk.

This walk didn't appear to be clearing my mom's head the way she had intended it to, though. As I tried to keep pace with her, she continued to complain, her face swollen and red, and her comments inched closer to actual rage. I had never seen her like this. She started talking about the double-standards for women, how they hurled themselves at the unbreakable glass ceiling.

Like when I was your age, I'd get groomed for these jobs, my mother said. Executive jobs. But blustery young men, wet behind the ears, would enter the company, and then I'd get passed over for positions that were rightfully mine. The management would give these coveted appointments on silver platters to these guys who had no experience at all. Eventually, the smooth-talking newbies would end up quitting anyway, because they had a cocaine problem, or a marital problem, or they had another job waiting somewhere else. Do you realize I went back to work when you were only two weeks old? TWO weeks for Chrissakes, she said. There I was, out in the bullshit world, my tits still leaking milk, washing out blood from my pantyhose in the bathrooms at work. But I was not going to leave the workplace because I wanted a better life for my family.

I tried to calm my mother down, insisting that she had made that better life. She started her own business, and she was officially my dad's boss—what could be more feminist than that?

This only seemed to make her angrier. The women of your generation haven't picked up the baton my generation passed you! she said, a choking snag appearing in her voice. The war isn't over, goddamnit! I need you to continue to fight!

Then she started to break down in a sob. All of those sacrifices, she said, I would never have made those sacrifices. If I knew I was going to be passed over like that, I would've stayed home with my baby because you never know when your baby is going to be sick, and when your baby is going to need you.

I realized this wasn't about all womankind anymore—it was about me. My mother had tried to keep me safe since the day I was born, and now she had to hand me over to someone else, to some male surgeon whom she didn't know, and had never been especially kind to us either. Qualified or not, it was not an easy transfer of power. If she could have done the surgery herself, she would have. My mother wiped the running snot off her face with her sweatshirt and I leaned in close to comfort her.

Mom, I whispered. Mommy. I think it's going to be okay.

Oh, it *is* going to be okay, she said, finally calm again. She kissed me and held me close: It will be okay because I say so.

Jonah told me he planned to treat me to any pre-op activity I wanted, though he was surprised I decided on horseback riding. He didn't know I liked horses at all, probably because there was never an opportunity to show him back in New York. But when my grandmother still lived in Montana, horseback riding was always the highlight of the trip for me. I knew that my motor skills or eyesight could be compromised as a result of this surgery. Maybe I'd never be able to ride again. It was the perfect gift. As we took a trail through Griffith Park, Jonah was enthusiastic to share a bit of research he learned as he was reading up on craniotomies.

Did you know, Lauren, that surgeries to the gut have much higher mortality rates than brain surgery?

I sighed. Jonah?

Yeah?

That's not incredibly helpful, trying to guide him to a social cue.

Oh. First he looked defeated, and then mortified. I don't know what

I'm doing really . . . I just thought you might think of it as some encouraging news.

And in a certain way, it was.

I appreciate the sentiment, I replied. I really do. But when people go in for an intestinal surgery, they don't have to fear that they are going to wake up an entirely new person.

Understood, he said. Sorry.

We touched hands briefly before my horse trotted ahead of his.

My legs gripped the saddle, my jeans drenched in sweat, but I didn't have to wrangle with the horse at all—it knew its way. At least someone did. And when Jonah rode up next to me, I asked him to do me a favor.

Anything, love, he said. Name it.

Can you bring a tape recorder to the hospital? I would ask my parents, but don't want them to have another thing to worry about.

He said it was an easy request and he would be happy to get one for me. But do you mind telling me why? he asked.

I mentioned the stories people had told me about what I was like after my first surgery. But they didn't always correspond with one another, and they didn't match some of my own personal recollections. And I didn't produce any audio recordings then. So if I had to go through all of this a second time, I wanted a more objective mediating force in the mix.

I see. He nodded and smiled. A woman after my own heart.

THE SIX STEPS OF A CRANIOTOMY

1. **Prepare the patient**

   No food or drink after midnight the day before. Not like you will be able to eat anyway. You won't be able to sleep either, even with your boyfriend in your bed. He will wake up when you wake up, and cradle you in his taut arms, but he will fall asleep soon after that with the ease of someone who won't be going under the knife the next day.

   Your younger sibling and his redheaded doppelgänger will be asleep when you leave in the early morning. But your brother will have given you a proper send-off the night before. He will have hugged you and offered you reassuring words, and you'll recognize how these earnest expressions have been lifted straight from your own glossary, things you said to him years ago as a toddler with a skinned knee, as a fifth grader taunted by a classmate. You'll be impressed by the ways your brother is turning into a kind man. Your boyfriend will come with you and your folks to the hospital, bringing the tape recorder you requested.

The nurse will check your blood pressure. She'll ask you to take a pregnancy test, too. You realize that all of your towering preparations for this day can be undone by pissing in a cup, so fingers crossed.

Before the general anesthesia, the paperwork you have been expecting will be set before you. And you will probably write in "Catholic" on the formerly vacant line. Then, you'll get your IV.

You'll be asleep before your head is put into a three-pin, skull-fixation device. Since all brains float in cerebral spinal fluid, a lumbar drain will be inserted to release some of that liquid to let the brain relax.

2. **Make a skin incision**

   Your scalp will be prepped with antiseptic, and a little past your hairline, an incision will be made. The surgical team will remove about a quarter of an inch of the hair around the site. Often, half of the scalp is shaved, and sometimes all of it, though female patients are occasionally treated differently than their male counterparts on this point. But this decision is purely cosmetic, and up to the discretion of the surgeon.

3. **Open the skull**

   The skin and muscles of your head will be folded back from the bone. A machine will drill into the cranium, creating one, or several, *burr holes*. A bone saw called a *craniotome* will cut a curved section of bone. When this bone flap is removed, the outermost layer of the brain, the *dura*, will be visible.

4. **Expose the brain**

   With a pair of surgical scissors, the operating team will pull back your dura like peeling the skin off of an overripe plum. Holding back surrounding brain tissue, *retractors* will be true to their name, as they isolate the area of interest.

5. **Correct the problem**

   A brain is a sloshy product inside an inflexible container. The compact surgical arena of the skull will limit all of your doctors' actions. The brain surgeons will wear magnifying gear over their eyes. They'll manipulate instruments with long handles and tiny tips. Everything is done in miniature in this work, like a Fabergé artist building a palace inside of an egg. Your surgeons will attempt to pass through this terrain without disturbing it too much, since there is always the risk of another rupture. Even in the surgical world, aneurysm interventions are often compared to defusing a bomb.

   Your aneurysm will be resting on the Middle Cerebral Artery, and the surgeons will take a metal clamp and try to close off the opening of the aneurysm. For the next second or two, they'll have to watch for the artery's response to this device. The surgeons will hope the clamp will fit there, because if not, they'll have to try something less orthodox, and perhaps less permanent.

6. **Close the craniotomy**

   People have been cutting into skulls for centuries, and not just in aggression, but in kindness, too. Sometimes it was thought that the easiest way to release the demon, the wandering spirit, the evil air, was to create an opening through the head and just let it out. These trepanations extend into the prehistory of the human race and their visible marks and gaping holes remain on the bones left behind. The vast majority of craniotomies do not leave openings in the skull anymore, though. Sutures will close the dura and the surgeons will return the bone flap to its initial location, securing it with plates and screws. But this closure will be carried out whether or not the problem has been corrected.

PART FOUR

UNFINISHED

I never lost as much but twice,
And that was in the sod.
Twice have I stood a beggar
Before the door of God!

Angels—twice descending
Reimbursed my store—
Burglar! Banker—Father!
I am poor once more!

EMILY DICKINSON

1

Morphine was dragging through my veins as I tried to make out the shapes before me. Two figures stood in front of a bank of windows, but the blinding sunlight streaming through made it impossible for me to look into their faces. I knew that they were my doctors only by their voices—Dr. Giannnota and Dr. Teitelbaum. The surgery was all done, and they were telling me that it had gone pretty well, considering. But very early on, the procedure had encountered a major complication.

I knew the doctors wouldn't try to remove the existing coils in my aneurysm because that operation had been deemed too dangerous ahead of time. But relying on the recanalization was a key component to the surgery they did plan. The coils were expected to have compacted farther into the aneurysm, so a metal clip could be easily fastened across the loose "neck" of the structure. However, once the surgeons had opened up my skull, they discovered the aneurysm was not as pliable as they'd hoped. There was not enough material to clip the structure closed. So, they had to improvise. Instead of clipping the aneurysm, they wrapped it—a rare procedure, but they had some experience with it. Careful to maintain the coils inside the structure, they coated the outside of it with cotton and superglue.

It was shocking to hear the material list, like an arts and crafts project filling my skull. My papier-mâché aneurysm.

I had prepared to ask the surgeons certain questions when I woke up. "How long will I be in the hospital?" And "Will I have to return to speech therapy?" Instead, though, I asked something that hadn't been part of any prepared list beforehand:

Will I still be able to have children one day?

Can't see any reason why not, Dr. Giannota said. Characteristically, his statement was blunt, and it was clear this topic didn't interest him in the slightest.

I am told that my parents came to my bedside in this period of slow awakening. Jonah too. When the drugs wore off and I was much more alert, I wanted a sense of how my spoken language had fared. Everyone told me I sounded fine, but I wanted to hear it for myself. So the day after the surgery, Jonah honored my request and turned on a tape recorder. *Click.*

ME: Hey, it's me.

JONAH: Then it's recording now . . .

ME: Oh. Well hello hello. It's me and Jonah.

JONAH: Hello.

ME: We are at USC. I'm up on my feet. I've seen my scar. It is disgustingly badass.

JONAH: It is wicked.

ME: It is very wicked. Uhhmm. My speech seems pretty good.

JONAH: It seems great.

ME: It seems great. Uhhmm. I don't know. What else can I tell you? My speech seems great. My, my head . . . I wore some blood around my, my chest for a few hours. They have just taken it away and Doctor Schmieeeeekaliebop just gave me an extra stitch. As he was doing that. Now I am wearing a very chic beanie. Anything to say?

JONAH: Uhh, I think you're doing great. You're better than I thought
          you'd be. Mmm, yep.

(A rustling sound and mutual laughter)

ME: He grabbed my butt.

It was the still hour after dawn and a nurse had unhooked my IV, promising to return in a few moments to take me on a walk down the hall. After
a few minutes, I heard a knock at the door. I got out of bed, impressed with
the strength and the evenness of my gait. But to my surprise, it wasn't the
nurse who greeted me. It was a priest.

He had a barrel chest and his black clerical shirt pulled at the paunch
near his midsection. He was balding, with a resilient ring of white hair
covering the final third of his head. With a crooked nose and unsmiling
lips, he had the look of a boxer. Or Dick Cheney. His heft was blocking
the doorway.

Good morning, he said. Would you like to receive the sacrament?

I felt I had received several sacraments already. It was a sacrament to
wake up from surgery. It was a sacrament that I could clearly read the
calendar on the wall; in fact, I was hugely grateful I could read anything.
I hadn't developed any visible seizures, and there were no traces of visual
deficits. And, most important, I was still able to write. What sacrament was
I meant to receive now?

Sorry? I asked. Could you explain what you mean?

Communion, he said. Would you like to receive Holy Communion?

Hmm . . . I considered. You know, I don't think so. But I can't thank
you enough for coming to see me!

To this day, I am not quite sure why I turned the priest away. A sense
of gratitude and sanctity was abounding in those moments, so why didn't
I want to receive communion from this holy man? If I hadn't survived the
operation, this was more than likely the cleric who would've administered
my last rites. I suspect if one of the missionaries from my neighborhood

had arrived at my hospital door instead and asked me the same question, I would have happily accepted the invitation. However, this priest had the face of a brawler, and I was in no mood to fight.

As his loafers clomped away, my aching face cracked into an uneven smile. I saw my reflection in the window—my lips were even on both sides of my face. Just another of today's sacraments.

2

Fewer than three days after I was admitted to the hospital, I was discharged. My parents and I were astonished. Jonah was still in town, and we were overjoyed we could spend more time together before he returned to New York. He was very careful with my face. My entire head was a tender coloring book. I had developed a tremendous black eye with splotches of green around it. There were blue lines from the surgical markings, and a red scar pulled together with jagged black stitches. The surgeons had shaved only around the incision point on my head, leaving me the vast majority of my hair. This was all hidden under a beige cap that the hospital had given me, and eventually, the whole thing could be easily disguised with an artful comb-over. But it itched like hell.

My first night home, Jonah and I climbed into bed in my newly red room. The equanimity I had felt in the house before the operation was not exactly holding fast. With six adults on one floor, the quarters were feeling a little tight. Jonah and I were sharing the unlockable bathroom with the Michaels, and the area was showing the general disorder produced by two boys in their twenties. But I liked that the two were bonding. From time to time I overheard Materson asking my brother for tips on picking up American girls, and in turn, Mike had confided in Materson about his issues with Amber, hoping to get some insight from a fresh perspective. It was nice they were getting along. That being said, they also went to bed late and woke up late, and tended to slam the bathroom door at all hours.

After a particularly vigorous slam of that door one night, Jonah did not try to disguise his annoyance.

Your brother is a real piece of work, he said.

Tried to tell you. I laughed.

Jonah didn't. I was with your parents in the hospital all day when you were in surgery, he said. But neither of the Michaels showed up. They didn't make an appearance at all, even in the recovery ward. And when we all came back to the house, those slackers were on the couch watching TV.

Typical. I continued to smile, and shook my head. Now you know what I've been dealing with!

Jonah remained unmoved, though. When we returned from USC, I gave them the evil eye, he said, and that finally got them motivated. Or shamed them into submission.

Well, they got there eventually, I said, pulling back the covers and climbing into bed. That's what counts.

Does it? Jonah asked. I know that Scottish kid probably can't drive in the US, but your brother should have known better.

It's not a big deal, I said, surprised Jonah was still focusing on this.

I sort of think it is, Lauren. Your brother should have been there for you, and he just wasn't. He really dropped the ball.

This comment brought out a mixture of emotions from me. It was sweet that Jonah was being protective, but I thought he was also being much more judgmental than necessary. He hadn't even gotten into bed with me yet, and at this point, there was a coastline of pillows separating us.

They are just kids, I said, hoping to defuse his mood. Don't you think you might be overreacting a little?

To tell you the truth, he snapped, I think you might be *under*reacting.

•   •   •

What Jonah was not emphasizing was the fact that the Michaels did eventually arrive that day. It was just when everyone else had left, and visiting hours were long over. The windows of the ward were black, with only dim working lights on the floor, so when a nurse came over to me, her voice was like a tiptoe. I only heard every other quiet word, but was able to make out, *brothers* and *exception*. Then a broad blur of red appeared, flanking me on both sides of the bed.

Can't believe that worked! Materson whispered gleefully. We had to fib a little to get in at this hour, but Mike gave an Oscar-winning performance! Told the nurse that we were both your brothers, both in from Scotland. And he put on this rubbish accent, too, but somehow fully convinced the staff that our flight came in late at LAX.

I had it under control, Sis, Mike said. You know I would have done anything to get to you.

My brother looked like a man who had been camping for days, with disheveled hair and a spotty three-day beard. Then he started to take off layers. First one bag, then another. On a nearby chair, he deposited his keys, pens, matches, Zippo, gum, and then his jacket. He was an urban sherpa setting up base camp. He was making himself lighter and I was feeling lighter because of it. He held my hand and kissed the part of my face that wasn't swollen.

Love you so much, Sis. Mike breathed out heavily. So glad you are okay. And I squeezed his hand. This visit couldn't have gone better if I had planned it.

My brother's intentions are good, I told Jonah. They are just not always visible. My eyebrows wrinkled, an action that I wasn't usually conscious of, but this time I could feel that the left side of my brow was still leaden and sluggish.

Well, I think your brother needs to take responsibility for his actions, and his inactions, too. It seemed to me that Jonah was trying to emphasize his point because he stood in his underwear on the cold wood floor instead of climbing under the covers with me. Mike's not a kid anymore, he said.

Now I sat straight up myself. But he is still my *kid* brother, I said.

It was only then did I realize Jonah and I perceived this situation in fundamentally different ways. I knew my brother often got uncomfortable in hospitals, and I hadn't expected him to leap into action when I was going into surgery. It wasn't at all a surprise that he procrastinated until the last possible minute, and, regardless, he had gotten to me.

There were decades I had shared with Michael that I still couldn't access in detail. But I knew intrinsically that before the stroke I often took on a custodial role with him, and I also knew that the roles had largely reversed over the last several months. Yet even in my most detached states, it was abundantly clear to me that even though the bond between us had changed, it had never disappeared.

Mike is very invested in what is happening around him, I said to Jonah. He's emotional—sometimes overly so. If he looks disinterested, it's usually a defense because he gets overwhelmed.

You might be right, Jonah said, finally getting under the covers. But what I saw today was a man who doesn't care about anything.

Then you missed it, I said, now too agitated to drift off to sleep.

It seemed that Jonah didn't understand my family at all, or the particular ways we expressed our affection. I felt I needed the final word before I turned off the lamp that night, and I tried to gather the most specific language I could muster.

It's not that my brother doesn't care, I told Jonah. He can't help himself from caring. He cares without abandon and without being able to stop caring about everything and everybody. Like most of my family members, I said, he probably cares a little too much.

3

As I flipped through the hefty packet of documents I had been given upon my release from the hospital, it was immediately clear that it still wasn't comprehensive enough for me. Was I sleeping on the scar correctly? What kind of pressure should I be applying or avoiding? How long did I have to wait before taking a shower? Should the screws be protruding from just below the skin that way? There were just enough rules to keep me out of serious danger, but not enough to help me minimize it during everyday life.

Mike had returned to Monterey. Jonah had returned to New York. Materson, making the most of his gap year, was off to the Bahamas. I had the house to myself again, and I spent hours soaking in the bath, usually wondering about the proper maintenance of my head. Going through so much trouble and expense, I didn't want the work to be undone by something as ridiculous as using hair gel too early or picking the itching scar. I needed to talk to a professional. Luckily, my post-surgical consult with Dr. Giannotta was scheduled for later that week.

Dr. Giannotta's tie was comic-book blue. His beige slacks and loafers screamed Clark Kent, but the tie, with its geometric patterns and glimmering metallic sheen, was all Superman. He was satisfied with the way the incision was healing, and said I'd have a checkup in July. Another angio-gram. Then he went through my questions one by one.

He said it was safe to exercise again. And if I wanted to return to yoga soon, I shouldn't do headstands or handstands for the next three months.

When can I cut my hair?

In a couple of weeks.

Can I get on an airplane now?

No one is stopping you.

And what about roller coasters?

Are you kidding me right now? he asked. After all this? His face was so impassive and I couldn't tell if he was teasing me or not. Grow up, he said.

It was the professional opinion of the surgical team at USC that I had undergone two "unfinished" operations—the one in Scotland and the one in Los Angeles.

They called them "unfinished" because neither one had accomplished what they had set out to do. After the first intervention, the coils had even-tually drifted from the walls of the aneurysm, and during the second in-tervention, the surgical clip couldn't be set in place. There wasn't enough research on cases like mine to know what came next—very few people had wrapping on top of coiling—so in many ways, my operation had been successful, but my "success" was conditional. There were two aneurysms in my brain, one that had ruptured and been treated, and another that hadn't. When an unruptured aneurysm remains in the brain, its risk of rupture increases by .05 percent per year. I certainly didn't want any more surgeries in my life, but it would always be a possibility.

And though my language had not been further damaged in the sur-gery, I still had my lifelong aphasia to attend to, whatever that might mean.

In an immediate sense, though, I had never paid so much attention to my head. I kept running my fingers over my skull, exploring the terrain that had been added by the surgery and what had always been there. I was like an amateur phrenologist.

Phrenology is the analysis of the bumps and ridges of a person's head, a practice meant to deduce inherent traits and abilities. Now debunked as a pseudoscience, there is no legitimate scientist who would trust in the analytic skills of phrenology these days. But the knowledge we have regarding the function and dysfunction of the brain didn't come to us on a straightforward line. And, in fact, many important figures of modern day neuroscience openly acknowledge the debt their discipline owes to phrenology.

Franz Gall, phrenology's founder, was a physician and anatomist who sincerely believed there was a direct correlation between the cranial topography and the actual functions inside the brain. In the early- and mid-1800s, the medical profession considered this approach to be a viable diagnostic tool, and presidents and poets alike consulted phrenologists worldwide. Gall said that the more pronounced the activity in the brain, the more it will be visible on the skull itself. Though this theory was later disproven, it did have significant influence in a sidelong way. Roughly sixty years after the heyday of phrenology, a Canadian neurosurgeon named Wilder Penfield was conducting brain surgeries on patients who needed to be awake so he could accurately pinpoint the source of their disturbances. As a result of this intricate and unprecedented work, he was able to observe which parts of the brain generally controlled which parts of the body. Unlike the phrenologists, who had mapped the outside of the skull, Penfield started to map the inside of it—and he produced something that is still referred to as the *Penfield Map*. This was a phenomenal leap forward for neuroscience. The brain was divided into specific quadrants, and as scientists started to assign certain functions to these locales, this approach to the brain took on the name *localization*.

There were early detractors against the purely localized model that Penfield proposed. Marie-Jean-Pierre Flourens, Jules Cotard, and Sigmund Freud (who was still a young neurologist in Vienna) all voiced their concerns. But they were voices in the wilderness. The prevailing view had become that the brain was overtly mechanical, with a single location, single function model. And although this idea reinforced the discoveries of the language centers by Broca and Wernicke a few decades earlier, it was often disastrous when doctors considered brain patients like myself. The whole principle suggested that the broken parts of us could never be repaired.

It took more than a century to allow for a more flexible approach to the brain to be taken seriously. In the 1960s, Paul Bach-y-Rita was already an esteemed scientist with expertise in medicine, neurophysiology, and psychopharmacology. His father suffered a debilitating stroke in 1965, losing his ability to use half of his face and body and some language. Very slowly, and with a lot of assistance, his father recovered many of his former capacities, eventually able to return to teaching at the university level and do some mountain climbing, too. Since brain scans did not yet exist, it was only after his father's eventual death years later that Paul Bach-y-Rita was able to appreciate what had actually happened in his father's recovery. A colleague of his had done his father's autopsy and insisted that Bach-y-Rita look over something totally unexpected in the brain sample. He was very reluctant to examine any part of his father's remains, but suddenly realized why he was being consulted about the matter. If following a localization model, this kind of large-scale recovery could only happen if the senior Bach-y-Rita had never sustained very serious damage to his brain initially. But that was not what the young Bach-y-Rita was seeing under his microscope.

In Norman Doidge's *The Brain That Changes Itself*, Paul Bach-y-Rita explains, "Major brain centers in the cortex that control movement had been destroyed . . ." adding there still was, "a huge lesion from his stroke and that it had never healed, even though he recovered all those functions." This sparked a revelation in the scientist, who says that in this moment he became aware that his father's brain "had totally reorganized itself." These changes in synaptic connections and neural pathways, which could then manifest as changes in behavior and ability, challenged the very idea of the organ as immutable. This perspective of the brain came to be referred to as *neuroplasticity*.

To be very clear on this point—localization and neuroplasticity are not mutually exclusive. Localization provides the most basic understanding of the brain/body connection. And neuroplasticity shows the ways in which flexibility can be inserted into these systems.

It is likely that I was the beneficiary of many neuroplastic changes throughout my recovery. That would mean that some of the speech and language areas of my brain were actually destroyed in my injury, and nontraditional areas of the brain took on their workload. But even though there have been tremendous advances in the years between Bach-y-Rita's stroke and my own (including the advancements of several types of brain imaging), even the most sophisticated scans can still fall short. If someone wanted to accurately track the neuroplasticity in a single person, the most optimal way would be to have brain imaging made before and after a stroke, for a real basis for comparison. But since strokes are often unexpected, this is very rarely possible.

For a variety of reasons, I have never been able to adequately discover the extent of the neuroplastic changes in myself—or, at least, as they might appear on brain scans. This means I can only ask questions in a more broad, philosophical sense, like: Why would I have continued to improve after the ruptured aneurysm when so many people in the same situation do not?

And I think the answer to such a question is probably quite layered. First, the speed of my initial treatment was key, in addition to the fact that I was cared for by medical professionals with the highest level of expertise. Second, the support of my family was invaluable, affording me ample space and time for my rehabilitation. Third, I was younger than many stroke survivors, which has its own recuperative advantages. And some specialists I have consulted with over the years have even speculated that my background in performance or academia, or both, might have contributed to an unusual skill set that I could draw on as a hidden resource, like a cognitive reserve. Or maybe my injury was never that profound in the first place? But as far as I can tell, there is no way to test this.

As a discipline, neuroscience is still only in its earliest stages. This means that I will always have many unanswered questions about myself. Even though I was taking authority over my own body after the craniotomy, and slowly taking control of the ways I might be able to analyze my progress with my language disorder, this didn't change the fact that I could not know what was actually happening inside of me on a cellular level. Could never know. And actually, I find that a little delightful. Perhaps it will only be a neuropathologist, handling a few slices of my lifeless brain, who will be the first person to understand what progress really meant in a case such as mine.

4

In the weeks after the surgery, I got to work thanking everyone who had been reaching out to me. At the end of every note, I drew a sketch of myself with my stitched horseshoe scar. I thought the cartoon was cheerful, but my mother told me that some people might find the drawing a little ghoulish, so I went back to signing my name instead.

BJ called me midtask and asked how I was adjusting to life outside of the hospital.

It's normal, I guess. Everything is incredibly normal out here.

You sound disappointed! he said. What were you expecting?

I wasn't at all disappointed—my relief was beyond measure. But it was odd to be on the other side of this surgery. My parents and I had spent so much time fixating on it, preparing for it, and now it was simply over and we had been spared all the possible catastrophes we had steeled ourselves for. My cousin Spencer was improving, too. He had been the center of widespread family concern after partially shattering some of his vertebrae on his spinal column in an off-roading motorbike accident many months ago. Like my parents had done for me in Scotland, his father had moved in with him to help with the rehabilitation. After undergoing an experimental neurosurgery on his spine, he was walking again, and he impressed everyone when he returned to work. But progress was slow. I didn't know how Spencer was dealing with his own medical concerns and—in spite of our strangely similar experiences—I hadn't reached out to him.

Our family was relatively small, and for several years, Spencer and I were the only grandchildren in it. I suspect our neurological struggles were too overwhelming, and too internal, to even think about reaching out to each other in the months after our injuries. But he would be visiting LA in a few weeks for business. If I wanted to, I could ask him about his life post-injury in person.

But when it came to my own body, it was hard not to feel strangely adrift.

How is your family doing post-craniotomy? BJ asked. Decompressing?

Not exactly. I laughed. They've just moved on to other minor crises.

Does this mean you are ready to come back to New York? He sounded hopeful. Not trying to rush you. But, I mean, what happens now?

It was something I had to consider.

The Girl I Used to Be had built up a life for twenty-seven years. The Woman I Was Becoming had only eight months under her belt. And these two lives existed in patches and scraps, divided in separate heaps, on two different coasts. Maybe now it was time to lay all the material out in front of me, to see what could be sewn together, and what would be discarded.

Following the Scottish procedure, everything I did had been focused on the immediacy of my medical and therapeutic interventions. Speech therapy, language rehabilitation, even the craniotomy. It had all been putting out fires. The period after the second surgery didn't have to be so reactive but proactive. My spoken language was better, my ability to read was improving, which meant my capacity to learn and synthesize more information was promising, too. The surgeon had warned that I might make a significant linguistic backslide as a result of the operation, but I expressed my glee of proving him wrong in my journal.

I was able to write much before the surgury. ~~There~~ In writing, there is some amount of remedy and there is another amount of poison. But here I

am. Lucky again. Sentences, and paragraphs, at the ready. I didn't ~~know~~
I what would happen in the surgery, in the percentiles? Lose language, lose
my life? But I woke up on started cussing up a storm.

But it became clear that the path forward required looking back a bit.
It seemed that whatever I wanted to pursue, I might benefit from knowing
more about what had already taken place in my life. What could I still do,
and how could I do it? Could I ever return to the life of The Girl I Used
to Be? And would I even want to? I took a quick physical inventory. . . .

Today (2 weeks since brain surgery)

- *still no period (8 months)*
- *no job, no swchool, no apt*
- *a scar from ear to mid forehead*
- *a sliver of blood in my L eye*
- *not much super glue on my scalp*
- *a tingling plump lip (sexy. plus)*
- *no swimming*

What happened now? I wondered. The psychic inventory was not so
easy. There was such an enormity in that question that I wasn't able to even
approach yet, but I did scratch out the first and only idea that came to my
mind:

start the memoir.

APRIL

APRIL

5

It was the first Wednesday of May, which meant that the peace and justice workers across the street would be meeting for oatmeal. Though most of the members of the group hadn't seen me since the surgery, my neighbors, Russ and Gloria, had checked on me soon after the operation, a little surprised when I had answered the door myself. They handed me some cupcakes and I assured them the black eye wasn't as painful as it looked. I promised them I would be at their next meeting. It had become somewhat of a ritual for me. When I walked through the door on the day of my return, I was quietly congratulated on the surgery's success. But the attention did not last for long. Today's focus was Bob.

Bob was one of the senior members of the group, who had come in that day with his wife. Between passing berries and multi-grain toast, I noticed how everyone in the room was tailoring their stories to Bob. How they met him, how his service had inspired their own. They talked about the variety of ways he changed the courses of their own missions. I went into the kitchen to refill the creamer, and Gloria snuck in to chat with me.

We should have prepared you for this beforehand, she apologized. Bob has been with us for years, and his health has been declining pretty dramatically. He's not long for this world. And . . . well . . . we all wanted to do a little something for him, you know? To celebrate his life.

It was a living wake. The whole thing reminded me of the e-mails people had sent to me in Scotland, which my parents had read aloud. There were plenty of notes of admiration or encouragement. But a lot of other e-mails had a kind of finality to them, as if it might be the last time the letter writers would ever be able to reach out to me. There was one from my first love, Jason, a lush assemblage of our two years together—the avocados we ate, the art we admired, the ways we once planned to discipline our future children when they were bad. He mentioned that our relationship wasn't always perfect and it hadn't ended well, but we had laughed a lot, and more than anything, we were each other's first loves. No one could take that away from us.

The letters were unusually direct. As people, we don't often face one another and explicitly say: you have made an impression on me. My life is different, and better, for knowing you. I hadn't appreciated the gift of these letters when they had been sent to me initially. It wasn't that I disliked hearing from people, but at the time, the memories they shared just did not elicit an emotional reaction in me. Later, though, I would come to treasure them.

Now, I wondered how Bob felt, with his friends around him, reviewing his life as they knew it. He was probably aware of why he was being singled out for this attention—was he annoyed or scared, grateful or curious? Was he indulging his inner Huck Finn, in the rafters of the church at his own funeral? I didn't ask. His wife told me that Bob's words had become fewer and fewer. Was it progressive aphasia, like Emerson? I tore out an empty journal page, jotted down the name of my speech therapist, and handed it to her.

Don't know if it would help, I said. But in case you need it. It was a small gesture, but it was the least I could do for the community for which I was so grateful.

I am an honorary grandparent. Mainly, Montday through Friday, I am alone in my attic. I when I do see people, I see old people. My Grandma

and her friends Or the member of the peace and justice group next door,
first Wednesday of the month. Most of those members have 30 years at
least on me. But grandparents ~~I know~~ and I have a lot in common. I
have our days to ourselves, filled with thoughts and tinkerings. ⧚ The
grandparents and I share stories of surgeries and share scars, actual and
metaphorical. Grandparents and I look a bit ~~i~~at the world outside with a
bit of bewilderment. The fray doesn't seem to miss us.

6

Usually, my grandmother spent her afternoons at the library. But this afternoon in May, she broke her routine to take a trip to the grocery store. It was of the highest priority because my cousin Spencer was coming into town.

Gram fussed about getting the right groceries. She wanted to pick up Spencer's favorite cereals and get the ingredients for his favorite meals, so I drove her to the market.

I don't want any bickering between you two, she warned me.

Why would we bicker? I asked.

She chuckled. Then she reminded me that while I had always been something of an aunt to my youngest cousins, Spencer and I were much closer in age, more like brother and sister. And she added that we had more sibling rivalry than Michael and I ever did. Maybe you've grown out of it, but you two could be holy terrors when you were kids, she said. You were each perfect on your own, but you'd develop this competitive streak around each other.

Grandma hung her cane on the wheeling cart, and leaned into the bar for support. When you were baking with me in the kitchen, lo and behold, suddenly Spencer wanted to learn to bake too. If Spencer was riding on the toy tractor in the yard, you wanted to get on it right away, even though you had ignored it all summer. And he would tell these harmless little stories about being in the CIA or FBI, which were ridiculous, since he was only seven years old. But Spencer's tall tales would just make you furious.

Really? I asked her, curious. This wasn't ringing any bells in my memory. Are you saying that I'd get angry with him?

That's putting it nicely. You'd both tattle on each other, and make me the referee. And in your ongoing attempt for competing for my attention as adults, you raised the stakes to dueling neurosurgeries! My grandmother gave me a tight pinch on my arm. Only teasing about that, punkin. It wasn't your fault this time, of course. But you little stinkers did give me the fright of my life last summer!

It had been years since I had seen Spencer in person, and when he arrived at Gram's door, I was amazed by how much he looked like my uncle, his father. His hair was more blond than brown, and tended toward corkscrew curls around his ears. Later that evening, we were sitting on the patio chairs in the backyard. Spencer was reluctant to go in, even in the waning light. In the part of Montana where our family had grown up, there weren't many days of the year one could sit comfortably outside. Winter was too long and too cold, and summer was plagued by swarms of mosquitos.

Spencer was bragging to me how his smooth talking had recently gotten him a used boat. This old drunk was asking five thousand dollars for it, Spencer said, but I bargained him down to one thousand and a bottle of Maker's Mark!

I had a twinge of envy listening to my cousin's story. Not about the boat—I couldn't care less about that—but his silvered-tongued power of persuasion. This was a trait Spencer and I used to have in common that was now almost entirely lost in me.

Spencer was leaving soon and I asked him if he was willing to show me his surgical scars, wanting to compare battle wounds.

His bare arms stiffened. All right, he said, though clearly uncomfortable. But only for you, Cuz.

He hiked up his T-shirt to the base of his neck. The incisions were fleshy white, hardened into a shape and color he would carry for the rest of his life. It was not just one scar, but dozens of them, like a bird's nest that had been pulled apart and then laid out over the length of his back. Then I showed him my scar, too, its pink and white tracks, from earlobe to forehead.

I'll be damned, he said, coming closer for inspection. It's almost exactly the size and shape of a horseshoe. It's like you are walking luck!

My cousin and I were still young, our faces mainly unlined. But peel off a shirt or remove a curtain of hair, and our scars could rival the worst of them. Looking so closely at each other was a bit like encountering a funhouse mirror. We were seeing very similar aspects of ourselves reflected between us, but we were also seeing aspects of the reality we only narrowly avoided. Watching how Spencer moved, it was clear he was still in pain; even sitting for him was difficult sometimes. And when he saw me, he understood a bit about my battle with my language and my memories. Our mutual admiration was infused with a guilty sense of gratitude. Though we had been spared a particular type of unpleasantness, someone we knew would have to bear it instead. And I think Spencer picked up on my slight jealousy, about how he was able to return to everything so much more quickly than me. So he compensated with a compliment.

Been meaning to tell you something, he said. I didn't see you right when the injury happened, but listening to you talk now, I have to say that your vocabulary is better than most people I know. Hell, he said, I think it's better than mine!

He was exaggerating again, this time for my benefit. And I appreciated it. There was such a thing as a helpful deception.

7

Jonah and I were chatting over the phone, and by the end of the call, he was trying to convince me to come back to New York earlier than I had initially planned. I was thinking about July, after my post-surgical angiogram. But he didn't want me to wait that long. Why not May? he asked. After some deliberation with my mother, we agreed on June.

Finally! Jonah said. Your triumphant return!

It was a funny bit of phrasing. *Return.* Was I *visiting* New York, or *returning* to it? Conversely, had I returned to LA? Or was that the place I had been visiting?

Regardless, Jonah's request had brought up the long-neglected issue of my New York home. I wasn't paying for school now that I wasn't attending it, but my apartment was another issue entirely. Before the aneurysm's rupture, I had shared my place in Greenpoint with an Australian journalist who was finishing his master's at NYU. But he had graduated and moved out while I was in California, and several of my friends had pitched in to help me find subletters. It was a sunny place, with a garden and a view of the Empire State Building, not to mention subway access on the corner— this profile itself made it somewhat easy to fill. But the tenancy was all short-term. In the course of nine months after the aneurysm's rupture, seven people had inhabited the two-bedroom flat, a few of them strangers; and two recent tenants had broken their agreement the month I was having the craniotomy. A generous acquaintance was staying in one of the rooms now, covering the majority of the rent, and my family was paying the remainder. My mother reminded me that she preferred that the situation be attended to sooner rather than later.

I'd leave after the first week in June and stay for three weeks. Though, try as I might, it was nearly impossible to cut and paste a version of myself in New York.

I planned to e-mail the current subletter, to ask if she minded if I stayed in the empty bedroom occasionally while I was there. But Jonah said there was no need.

That's silly, he said. You'll be living here in my place anyway.

Living here. It sounded so permanent. Perhaps he hadn't meant it that way, but months earlier, Jonah had said *Stay* here. His language had tweaked since then. Now he was saying: *Live* here.

talking with Jonah last night. twice he has more than hinted that he would want me to move in with him. but something feels misplaced. why would he want me to me to move in now—in my absence, and after years of ambiguity (I know I am changed and perhaps him too over the last year). I tell him I have difficulty reconcile myself to myself. My stories, my thoughts, my life, before the aneurysm.

It occurred to me then that in the years Jonah and I had spent as a couple in New York, we had never discussed living together. Jonah talking about it directly probably would have felt like progress to The Girl I Used to Be, proof that the relationship was taking a step forward. But with no clear sense of my own direction, the prospect of the three-week experiment was just a bit confusing for me.

Jo? I asked him. I know it might sound weird. But can you tell me a little more about our relationship? Can you tell me "the story of us?"

Though I remembered the big things, I wanted desperately to hear about little things. I remembered a lot of Paris. I remembered some of Scotland. I remembered plenty of Los Angeles, especially after the rupture. But there was so much still missing, especially from my time in New York, and a lot of that had been when Jonah and I had been together. After the second surgery, I felt a more urgent need to contextualize, to understand more about the life I used to inhabit. I had asked him versions of this question before, but this time I could tell he knew I needed him to take the request seriously.

Well. He hesitated. What do you want to know?

Everything, I said. I want to hear about everything.

Lauren, there is no easy way to answer this question, he said. And even if I could . . . well . . . there are some bits I don't want to relive. You know? There is a lot I'm not proud of.

I don't want you to feel bad, I said. Or embarrassed or whatever. The whole thing is so distant for me, so there is no way I can get upset. But I'm under the impression that our relationship was somehow . . . fraught? Like Michael and Amber.

First of all, we weren't anything like your brother and his hot mess, Jonah said definitively. But we did fall in love when we were really young. We were both smart and opinionated, so we challenged each other in good and bad ways. There was flexibility in our relationship, and I think I took advantage of that more than I should have. He sighed. But you were never a pushover. You could be tough as nails—it was one of the things I most liked about you. It was like you were the only person who could really take me to task. So, I think "the story of us" was a constant balancing act of intimacy and independence. Does that answer your question?

It started to, but I wanted hours and hours of more details. Like, if we were so opinionated, what had been the content of our opinions? What did we agree and disagree upon? I pressed him: What sort of things did we use to say to each other during our fights? I need some reminders from you. The more language I get, the more memories come back to me. . . .

Okay, Lauren. Jonah didn't seem angry or defensive at all, but his tone was a little worn down. I get what you are saying, and hear how important this is to you. So I want to help you out on this, I do.

But . . . He stopped himself. And after another moment of consideration, he continued, I just can't help but feel that rehashing this ancient history is a little counterproductive in a way. We've got an opportunity for a new beginning here? There are so many couples who really just want to reset the clock on their relationship, and you and I actually get that chance. And slowly, I think I am finally becoming the sort of person I should always have been for you. I understand that you want to talk about how we were, but I like how we are. Right now.

I do too, I said, and I meant it. But there was still so much I wanted to know, and since the ideas still lingered in my imagination, I continued to write about it.

I said, "What about are our story? How did it begin? How did it changed. What happened?" I tell him not to leave anything out.

He is retiscent. He doesn't want to talk about it, but is not angry either.

The question that hums
Or we better mates in absence then in presence?

When I had asked Jonah to remind me of the sorts of language we used in the last incarnation of our relationship, it was somewhat revisiting the topic of "linguistic relativity" that Jonah and I had started talking about soon after the rupture. Jonah had made clear his position on the matter: words didn't have a lot of bearing on perception, and language represented problems that exist, with or without words. But I still felt that language had a lot more agency.

In its "strongest" form, the Sapir-Whorf Hypothesis suggests that human beings are hugely constrained by language, both in thought and action. Its weaker form is more malleable, simply suggesting that language can have unexpected influences on behavior and thought.

But if language can actually change thought, how can that idea be tested? This is something that transnational scholar Lera Boroditsky explores in her work. Boroditsky came of age during a period of flux in the field of linguistics, and though the discipline is still influenced by theory, it now also includes rigorously controlled experiments whenever possible. She firmly believes that understanding linguistic relativity can give "fascinating insights into the origins of knowledge and the construction of reality."

Personally, I find Boroditsky's research most convincing when it is seeking out the effects of language in "seemingly nonlinguistic tasks." Like color tests.

Russian was Boroditsky's first language, but she is also an academic who operates fluently in English, which gives her a unique perspective on the differences between the two tongues. Boroditsky explains that Russian has no single word for the color *blue*. She writes, "Unlike English, Russian makes an obligatory distinction between lighter blues ('*goluboy*') and darker blues ('*siniy*'). We investigated whether this linguistic difference leads to differences in color discrimination."

The results of these tests were stunning. Boroditsky found that native Russian speakers were faster in color discrimination tasks, specifically "when they fell into different linguistic categories in Russian." Native English speakers could identify the subtle differences in color as well, but they were much slower. The Russian speakers had instinctual, habitual reactions. Their language training was "on-line" even when it seemingly should have been "off-line," and when they didn't need to think about language at all.

And Boroditsky and her colleagues have amassed dozens of tests like these, and they don't just deal with color and space, but sense of direction, too. They also explore the ways people perceive culpability and intentionality, from politics to the courtroom. Time and again, Boroditsky sees how language influences areas of our lives that are generally assumed to be nonlinguistic. Plenty of linguists disagree with this baseline, but even Steven Pinker, an outspoken critic of linguistic relativity in general, has written about Boroditsky as a persuasive figure. "She will be a force to be reckoned with," he writes, "even if I don't agree with everything she says."

I had not read Boroditsky this soon after the aneurysm's rupture, so I didn't have her research to cite when in discussion with Jonah, but she investigated a lot of issues I felt intimately connected with at the time. In my own limited way, though, I continued to tell Jonah that language hones many types of perception. I said that these perceptions affect the way we think about the world, and the way we are able to engage with it. It was unlikely that Jonah would ever fully agree with me on this point. But as Pinker had addressed the potency in Boroditsky's approach to linguistic relativity, Jonah was willing to cede some ground, too. He had come to realize the role language seemed to play for me, in activating some of my memories at least. So much so that he was reluctant to revisit the sorts of words we used with each other before the rupture, unwilling to disturb the spirits of our past selves.

And as a general principle, I saw that language required a focused attention from its speakers, which created an invisible skill set inside of them. We could never know the extent of those effects. The words we use, and don't use, could potentially permeate everything we do.

8

I picked Rachel up at LAX just before Memorial Day and brought her back to our house, where she would be staying for the California leg of her book tour. My bleary-eyed brother welcomed her at the door, and started to make her a breakfast of leftover pasta and scrambled eggs. Rachel had known Mike since he was a preteen, and they shared a sardonic and unflinching sense of humor that had only grown over the years. They started firing off movie and TV quotes in quick succession, mocking each other with inside jokes, inadvertently excluding me from the conversation entirely. I wanted to keep up and felt that I should have been able to—I was the person who had introduced them and had been in on all of those jokes once. But it took me ages to pinpoint what they were referencing, and when I did, they had already jumped to their next topic. So I hardly said anything at all.

Early in our friendship, Rachel and I were involved in a production of *The Bacchae 2.1*, Charles Mee's modern adaption of Euripides's Greek tragedy. We played the followers of Dionysus, known as the Bacchae. Rachel was the Lavender Woman, and I was the Orange Woman. Our characters were lovers, so we had to become physically and emotionally comfortable with each other pretty quickly during this production, and this show was mainly when she cemented her role as a permanent fixture in my group of closest friends. But neither of us was performing anymore. Rachel had mainly stopped acting by choice, and obviously I had stopped because of circumstance. And my aphasia made me doubt that I could ever be in a play again. Now that Rachel was on her first book tour, I was seeing how she had transformed herself from being an actor's actor, to a writer's writer. She had literally written herself into a new existence. The frenzy of her book tour brought out her most dazzling and manic energy. Her phone kept ringing—her managers, agents, editors, and publicity team. She barked at some of the people who called, squealed with glee with others. I was frustrated by the constant noise coming from her room. But ultimately, the speed and efficiency with which she managed these activities only illustrated how well she had taken to her new profession. My reactions to seeing Rachel in her element ran the gamut from admiration to jealousy. I sometimes thought of her like I did Casanova, changing all the aspects of her professional life, like she was just putting on a new skirt. She was a living testament that it was still possible to do that. But other times, I was stung by the nettles of desperation, because that sort of future seemed so out of reach for me.

If only I could remember my Orange Woman then, it might have given me some voice to my current sense of displacement. This woman stood bare-breasted before her audience every night agonizing over this sometimes mystifying, sometimes afflicting, quest for self:

My soul goes blindly seeking, seeking, asking.
Nothing answers.
I cry out after some unknown thing
with all the strength of my being
every nerve and fiber in my young woman's body
and my young woman's soul
reaches and strains in anguish.
At times waves of intense, hopeless longing rush over me,
my heart, my soul, my mind go wandering, wandering

groping with helpless hands
pursued by a demon of unrest
I shall go mad
I shall go mad
I say over and over to myself
but no.
No one goes mad.
The demon of unrest does not propose to release any of us.
He looks to it that our senses are kept fully intact.

So Spencer could get back to work, Rachel could be starting her second book, and I couldn't read a damn doctor's report. The interactions with these people close to me were fulfilling in so many ways, and their love for me was never in doubt, but being around them needled at me as well, because I was given an opportunity to measure out the vast distances between their lives and my own. It was my new demon of unrest.

9

It was difficult to understand what my brother was saying. It was still so early and I wasn't fully awake yet. As I pushed the phone closer into my ear, I heard him explain that Amber had been involved in a minor car accident. She was fine, but in pain and refusing to go to the hospital. Amber yelped in the background. Mike asked my parents if he could bring her home, and asked me if I had any leftover painkillers that might help. We all leaped into action.

My head was still tender, but I hadn't needed any of the codeine that had been prescribed since the operation, so I brought the bottle downstairs. My parents and I turned on the lights in the kitchen, all of us jittery, fearing a repeat of my brother's birthday. As Mike's car arrived, I heard Amber yelling at him from the driveway. Idiot! You fucking baby!

She took no notice of our assembled family as she slammed the back door open. The smell of alcohol on her was overpowering.

Mike carefully closed the door in her wake and looked up at us in shame.

I'm sorry, he said. I didn't know where else to take her.

Amber's eye makeup and lipstick were smudged across her face, her hair in a gnarl. Her left leg was visibly dragging. The foot on that leg displayed a scratched purple bruise, badly bandaged with toilet paper, which created its own train like an unraveling mummy. We tried to ask Amber what had happened, but she slumped on the far corner of the couch, continuing to ignore us, and cursed my brother again.

In a near stupor, Amber started to fish around in her purse until she found her phone. Her aggressive tone completely dissolved when someone picked up on the other side of the line—Mom? Amber asked softly. Mommy?

The new kindness of her voice was reflected in her face, too. She was small and plaintive. I saw a child's face emerging under that trembling lip. She was hurt, and she just wanted to come home. Would her mother drive across town and pick her up?

Instead, her mother hung up on her.

Devastated, Amber flung her phone onto the floor and let out a raspy moan. My mother grabbed some of the couch cushions to prop up Amber's foot, and placed an ice pack from the freezer on top of it. My dad picked out some ibuprofen, and whispered to me to put away my painkillers because it was dangerous with that much alcohol in her system. Mike got her water. While everyone tended to her, Amber continued to call him names. *Pathetic little faggot* was a term in heavy rotation. And I was seriously taken aback. Mike had told me Amber could get aggressive, but I had never heard it myself.

The tension in the room felt potentially explosive, and looking toward my parents, I sensed they felt the same way. But none of us said much. Not yet. Amber was in a furor, and no one wanted to change too many elements around her, for fear of an even more overwrought outpouring.

I thought of Rachel, who was sleeping in the room downstairs only a few yards away. She was a notorious insomniac, and I suspected she was overhearing all of this. There would be a lot to explain in the morning.

Amber was becoming less and less coherent, and while one part of me remained alert and attentive dealing with a woman in obvious pain, another part of me was relaxed. The tension, which had been building since my brother's phone call, had largely dissipated because of how he was behaving now. Amber was drunk, but Mike was sober. She was goading him, trying to send him into a rage, but he wasn't taking the bait. He sat in the armchair a few feet away, a little shell-shocked.

What a worthless piece of shit you are, she said to him. I mean, really. A total fucking waste of space.

It was just too much for me. A sudden, animalistic sense of protection overcame me. I grabbed for Amber's birdlike shoulders, and my reaction seemed to surprise both of us because she put up no resistance.

You are in pain and I want to help you with that. I do. But you are talking to my brother, who I love and will always love. I will help you with your damn foot, but only if I don't have to deal with your damn mouth.

Amber was stunned into silence, and though she briefly criticized my brother again—ironically this time saying that he should grow some balls like his sister—she passed out soon after that. Mike stood vigil as she drifted in and out of consciousness, replacing the ice pack when it slipped off her leg, and making sure she didn't choke in her sleep. He explained that he and Amber had been in a long and drawn-out breakup, and she had insisted they meet up to talk that night in a public space. She was already deliriously drunk when he arrived, and he decided he didn't want to engage with her like that. He got into his parked car and she threw herself on the hood, hurling her shoe at the windshield. And as soon as her feet were firmly back on the asphalt, Mike turned on the car to leave before the situation got any worse. This was when Amber appeared at the driver's-side window and started throwing punches. She knocked his recently lit cigarette out of his mouth, the glowing cherry dropping onto his jeans. As Mike described it, he didn't turn on the gas, but in an attempt to pat out the fire, his foot leaped off the brake on a reflex. And even without any speed behind it, the entire weight of the car rolled over Amber's bare foot.

Horrified that Amber might be seriously injured, Mike called 911 right away. But when emergency services actually arrived at the scene, Amber kept insulting the police officers and refused to get into the ambulance. The police attempted to interview them both, but my brother told me Amber had been too drunk to cooperate, and had continued to rant and rave. There had been CCTV footage recorded in that parking lot, allowing the police to confirm Mike's side of the story. They decided my brother was not at fault. No one was pressing charges and no one was being arrested.

I cringed when I heard that police had been called in the first place, wishing it had never escalated to that point, but I was glad of the resolution.

Did the police officers say anything else? I asked Mike.

Actually, yeah, he said, shaking his head. They said I should find myself a new girlfriend.

The next morning, my family continued to look after Amber—my brother and my grandma especially. Gram set up a makeshift nurse station for Amber by the couch with a bucket, washcloth, gauze, hydrogen peroxide, and a giant tube of Neosporin. When Amber woke up the first time, my grandma expertly cleaned the wound. It was unclear if Amber could remember the events of the previous night, or if she was pretending she didn't so she could save face. Either way, she interacted with all of us as if nothing out of the ordinary had happened. Then she fell back asleep. And when Rachel emerged from the spare bedroom, I discovered that she had actually slept through the entire thing. She was headed back to New York later that day, but with Amber snoring on the couch in the kitchen, we decided to go out to breakfast. Mike and my father stayed behind because they wanted to take Amber to have a proper checkup as soon as a doctor's office opened, but my mother was happy to get out of the house.

At Fox's Diner, my mother poured hot milk in the strong drip coffee. As we explained some of what had happened the night before, Rachel looked incredulous.

I can't believe that girl didn't try to sneak away when she sobered up a bit. Takes a lot of chutzpah not to slink out in the night or embark on her Limp of Shame in the morning, she said, looking at my mom. Suzanne, are you fine with this girl staying at your house?

My mom picked at her cinnamon roll with a single tine of her fork, exhausted. It's a balancing act with your children, she said. If you try to keep them away from something, or someone, they tend to run like hell in that direction. You've got to be as supportive as you can, and give advice only sparingly because if they marry a person they know you dislike, you'll become the enemy. Given a choice between partner and parent, your kids might choose partner instead.

Amber was hardly the ideal houseguest, but my mother refused to put her out while she was in pain, especially if she had nowhere else to go. My grandmother said almost the same thing. A doctor had examined Amber's foot and said that nothing was broken, but she stayed with us for several days after that. I started to grumble about her not needing us any longer—for a physically small girl, she took up a lot of psychic space. But it was my father and brother who insisted on her staying until Amber herself decided that she was well enough to go back to her house.

What kind of grace was it to have been born into a family like this?

If this was not a question I asked myself that morning, it was one I have asked many times since. My brother and I, I realized, had won the parental jackpot. When I had my stroke in Scotland, my parents had come running. I was lucky to have a family that had the desire, the resources, and the will to look after me. I was going through all of the stages of my life with them all over again, this time starting like a toddler. This was a somewhat accelerated course, and my parents provided but were also careful not to coddle. As they had done before my injury, my parents let me make my own discoveries, my own mistakes, without ever asserting an expiration date of their support. They were giving me the tools to forge a fierceness of mind again. I was close with my family before the rupture, but I suspect that The Girl I Used to Be didn't know how to manage this dynamic very well. She was neurotic, struggling to meet the demands of being a daughter and an older sister in such a close-knit family, while also wanting to fully differentiate herself from this powerful unit. Proof enough was the fact she moved three thousand miles away at her first opportunity. This time, my family members were coming to know each other as adults, and our dynamic was less like a hierarchy, more like an ecosystem. My mother and father had been willing to fly across the world when they knew their daughter was in danger. There were some parents who wouldn't drive across town. I didn't deserve these kinds of riches, but I knew I should appreciate it as long as I had them.

A few days later, after Amber had left, my own bags were packed, and I was almost completely ready to embark on my trip to New York. I was taking a break at the kitchen table, enjoying the warm breeze coming through the open windows, when my brother walked in. He double-checked that all of my suitcases were zipped.

Looks like you are all raring to go, Sis, he said. How are you feeling?

His words were incredibly simple, yet felt so extraordinary, that I couldn't say anything at all.

Earth to Lauren, my brother said, waving his arms in my direction.

Could you repeat the question? I asked.

Are you serious? he asked. All I asked was how you are feeling. . . .

Again, I paused. I often had to ask people to repeat a phrase, especially if they were saying a word or words I hadn't used since the rupture. Then I would try to mimic the unfamiliar sounds myself. This was totally different. People had asked me how I was doing, in this exact phrasing, ad nauseum. It had actually become white noise that I could tune out if I wanted to. But the phrase sounded newly minted when it was asked in my brother's voice.

I'm good, it's just . . . I stammered. I'm ready to head out, if that is what you are asking. But I'm having this strange experience, Mike . . . because I really can't remember the last time you asked me how I was doing. Was it before I left for Scotland?

Now it was my brother's turn for a brief silence.

Huh, he said. That's funny.

Am I wrong about that? I asked him.

Actually, I think you're right. Weird.

Well, if you haven't asked me that question before, why would you start now?

My brother said he needed a minute to think. Since I didn't realize I was doing that, he said, I might need a moment to formulate an actual response. One in which I don't sound like even more of a jerk . . .

After a short deliberation, he nodded to himself. Okay, he said. Okay. So when this whole aneurysm thing started, it was kind of a horror show. I had to stay with Grandma when Dad and Mom flew to Edinburgh. When the operation was over, and you were still in the hospital, I had to go back to college. I had no way to process what was going on. Didn't know who to talk to about it.

I'm sorry you were alone then, Mike, I said.

You shouldn't have to apologize. You of all people, he said. But I was in this total daze then. Doing everything on autopilot. And I blurted out that you had a brain aneurysm rupture to some random classmate, and totally without thinking about what he was saying, that guy told me that no one lives through that. Or if they do, they end up as human vegetables.

That's pretty offensive, I said. Not to mention factually incorrect . . .

Oh yeah, that guy is a total dick, he agreed. I knew he was a D-minus human even back then, but the threat took root with me. And when I did a little online research, everything seemed pretty bleak, so I couldn't motivate myself to keep looking. And even Amber told me to get comfortable with you dying, like it was an inevitability. Mike shuddered. Maybe that's the reason I never asked you how you were feeling. I probably didn't want a direct answer because you might say something I didn't want to hear. All the while, I just kept thinking that you still might die. You might die right in front of me.

He shook his head. I know my relationship with Amber has been bonkers for a long time—and I'm sorry you guys have had to endure some of that because of me. I know now that there is no chance we can stay together. But in this really, really small way, I think that part of the reason I kept trying to help Amber is because I couldn't help you.

I had never thought about it this way. In these months of confusion, while I had been worrying about my brother's safety and stability, he was worried about mine. And through a visibly dysfunctional relationship, he was also forging some well-earned resilience, and weathering more storms than I had realized. He was still experiencing growing pains, but I saw for the first time that he was emerging stronger on the other side. He was not someone I needed to care for in the way I used to; he was becoming someone who might occasionally care for me, too. He was making steps in that direction.

I reached for my brother's hand and apologized for the way I looked after the craniotomy, with the bloody eyes, the stitched skull. It had been out of my control, of course, but with that kind of fear stamped in his mind, it must have been so difficult for him to see me looking that battered.

Actually, no, he said. It was sort of great to see you in the hospital. And it's . . . it's all different now.

How? I asked. Why?

I can't tell you why, really. It's not exactly logical. After Scotland, you looked good, but sounded bad, and after this surgery, you looked worse but sounded better. And for some reason I can't exactly explain, I'm just not worried that you are going to die anymore.

Oh no? I asked.

No, he said firmly.

That's going to be hard to manage! I teased him a little. I can't promise I won't die ever, Mike. . . .

All right, he said. At some point, yes, you will. But not anytime soon. Mike leaned over and gave me a hug. I think you are going to be just fine.

10

In the second week of June, I headed to New York, hoping for a somewhat relaxing visit. But my social calendar had unexpectedly filled when word spread among my friends that I would be back in town. There were several people I had been in very sporadic contact with over this year, and others who had been the lifelines to my social life. BJ, Laura, Rachel, and Grace made sure we spent some quality time together. Jonah picked me up from JFK and brought me back to his apartment, carrying my suitcase up the three flights of stairs. While Los Angeles had already started its dry summer, New York was still mid-spring, the air crisp. Jonah sat down on the bed, while I looked in the direction of his crammed closet.

Is there space for my stuff in there too? I asked Jonah.

Oh, he said, still recovering his breath from the stairs. Um. You want to hang something up? Right now?

I nodded.

So Jonah quickly doubled up some shirts and freed a few hangers for me, but the space was too full for any new additions. He had a sturdy

1950s fan resting on a low bookshelf, and he ended up hanging a few of my dresses on its grate.

Sorry I hadn't thought about the closet space, Jonah said. That was a bozo move. I'm excited to have you here but I've never had any experience with living in the same room with someone else. Should I clean out a drawer for you too?

This lack of planning didn't rattle me much. Jonah's entire presence was welcoming; there was alertness in his eyes, affection in his touch, and just having his body near mine was a physical assurance of his care. I couldn't be numb to that. But it was disorienting to know that I had loved this person, in this exact place, but didn't really have any clear memories of doing so.

Jonah wanted me to feel like I belonged in his home, and I can't express what a genuine gift that really was since I wasn't sure of the person I was meant to be in New York. But whoever I was, whatever I was doing, I was not alone. When Jonah was being someone willing to provide this reassuring consistency, I felt a strong love for him. The love was largely disconnected from whatever we had before, though at least we were certainly still attracted to each other. However, if I was ever going to address the many points of my confusion with Jonah, it seemed I needed to know a lot more about the person he had fallen in love with.

I began by starting to re-familiarize myself with the apartment.

The place was small, but not by New York standards. And Jonah had cleaned for me. I noticed his bathtub and the black-and-white tile floor were both shining. The tiles underfoot were a little larger than pieces of a traditional mosaic, and when a few loose bits slipped as I stepped over them, I leaned over to replace them by hand. This gave me a powerful sense of tactile recognition. Not all memory retrieval is autobiographical. It can be procedural, too. Even people with profound amnesia, who cannot remember what happened a day earlier, or cannot encode new memories, either, remain able to learn new tasks. They can get better at puzzles, their proficiency improving day-by-day, regardless of whether they remembered seeing that puzzle before. Jonah's floor was a bit like that for me—tile and groove. I realized I had done this action many times before, though I couldn't remember how or when. This shape and this hand had most certainly met in this way many times over.

That bum landlord keeps saying he'll do something about it, Jonah said. And I'm sure he will. He'll just wait until I move out first.

The kitchen cupboards and fridge were almost bare. I had forgotten that Jonah ate out every day, a habit I couldn't afford to take up while I was here. I still had two brain surgeries to pay off. If I was going to cook in this apartment, I had to factor in the bare essentials. To make a salad, I'd have to buy a big bowl. To bake cookies, I'd need a cookie sheet.

I continued to wander. In this kitchen, there was a window that faced a dark airshaft, and resting against it were two cheap mirrors covered in paint. When I stepped a little closer, I realized they were two distinct characters. If I aligned my face correctly, a painted patch would cover my eye, a goatee would land on my chin, a spotted bandana would appear on my head, and a parrot would perch on my shoulder. And if I situated myself in the second mirror, I'd acquire a beauty mark, a Marie Antoinette inspired wig, and a glimpse of décolletage.

Gazing into these mirrors, I had another flash of recognition. I had painted these mirrors myself, and had given these to Jonah for some occasion or another. I found them funny, but a little creepy, too, because what kind of person would make a gift like this?

As I looked into my split reflections, I silently asked: *Who am I today? Pirate or queen?*

Since I came to New York. I am a dropped feather landed on this rushing city's river. Apt issues (moving out/, friends to catch up with/ and their shows to see, and staying at Jonahs house (instead of a room of my own).

I stayed in Brooklyn for five days before I even ventured out to visit my own apartment. When I finally got there, it was much worse than when I had seen it on my layover between Edinburgh and Los Angeles several months earlier. All I could do was survey the wreckage.

Grease spattered the walls of the kitchen. The doors were off the cupboards and the hinges were exposed. Pots and pans were littered across the floor.

There was no window in the bathroom, but the normally green-and-yellow tiles could have a sunny appearance, especially when the bathtub had been recently cleaned—which was clearly not today. The living room had been painted a sickly blue, an inconsistent coat that had been abandoned halfway through the job. The furniture had all been moved around. You couldn't see the garden or the Empire State Building from the couch anymore. In both of the bedrooms, there were piles of trash and clothes and electronics. My own bed had been hoisted on risers, affording a few more inches of storage space. But one of the blocks had been knocked off kilter, and hadn't been readjusted. My mattress looked like a sinking ship.

Before I went into the apartment, I had still been mulling over my tenancy options. Would I move back into this place at some point? Would I find another subletter in the meanwhile? This place had seemed a linchpin to my life on the East Coast.

But all my uncertainty vanished when I was physically in this space. My decision was neither conflicted nor sentimental. I wasn't sure where "home" was, but it certainly wasn't here.

11

My time with Grace was going to be much more limited than other friends—she had been offered a teaching position at Princeton that summer and was leaving town soon. She had suggested we have brunch near Morningside Park. This meant traveling all the way from Jonah's apartment deep in Brooklyn to upper Manhattan. She had no idea how bad I'd be at taking public transport, though. It was like I had never even visited the city before. I took too long at the MetroCard machine and was clumsy at the turnstiles, never able to adjust to the correct swiping speed for entrance. I held up lines, was cursed at, and was nearly trampled twice. I considered canceling our date, but pressed on. Not only did I want to see Grace, but she had a new boyfriend, too, an architecture student at Columbia, and she really wanted to introduce me to him. She thought he might be "the one."

The guy who now sat across from me at Max Caffé had a very calming energy. He was intelligent and engaging, but at some point in the conversation he stopped speaking to me entirely and appeared to be looking at the ceiling.

I assumed it was my fault. I was so out of practice with interactions, especially with strangers. I whispered to Grace and asked if I had done something wrong.

Grace laughed. She explained that her boyfriend was looking at the vents and ducts of the building, constructing its schematics in his mind. She said he often popped in and out that way, and I should definitely not take it personally. Before he resumed the conversation, she wanted to know what I was planning to do on this trip to New York. Had I visited my grad school yet? Seen any other friends?

I said I had to figure out my apartment issues first. I planned to see some friends' plays soon. But, more than anything, I was trying to write as much as I could.

Oh yeah? Grace asked. Are you still writing about the aneurysm?

I hesitated, recalling our last discussion about my writing in her parents' basement. Actually, I said, I think I am in the early stages of writing a memoir. Then I braced myself for a strident response.

That's fantastic! she said.

Really? I was surprised. You think it's a good idea? I sort of thought, because you didn't like the essay . . .

That's silly, Lauren. I knew it was important for you to write the essay, and I admired that you did. There was a lot I liked about it, too. I just had some concerns; some of them were legitimate, but a lot of them were motivated by my own worries. I was nervous about how this whole thing might be affecting our friendship. But a book about this experience is a great idea. It's the sort of thing that I would read, even if I didn't know you.

You would? I asked, instantly nourished by her enthusiasm.

Of course, she said. You should know my taste more than anyone.

It was a little embarrassing that I couldn't actually remember Grace's artistic likes and dislikes, but I knew that she and I had been talking about writing for more than a decade. Our years of friendship were suffused with language, from writing poetry side by side on Saturday mornings, to month-long discussions about our favorite books. Our freshman year of college, she had knitted me a scarf with a quotation from D. H. Lawrence's *Sons and Lovers*, a novel we had managed to both love and hate simultaneously. In black and blue yarn, she had stitched a line we had been obsessed with: *Like a creature awaiting immolation.*

This rich linguistic life that I shared with Grace had once been embedded in every interaction we had, braided into our familiar shorthand. But this mutuality had been all but erased in my stroke. How many friends had I abandoned this way—making them lone speakers of a now-extinct language? I thought about this when I met up with Grace, but even more later when I stumbled across two old instant message exchanges buried in my e-mail inbox.

The conversations were between the two of us, and though they were almost exactly the same length, the contents couldn't be any more dissimilar. The first interaction took place the day before the aneurysm's rupture. The second was eighteen days after it:

August 22, 2007, 2:03 pm

From:	GG
To:	LM
Date:	Wed, Aug 22, 2007 at 2:03 PM
Subject:	Chat with Grace G
mailed-by:	gmail.com

me:	hello
Grace:	hi hi

2:03 PM

me:	i am in scots land
	with kilts
	and bagpipes
Grace:	wow
	awesome
	i'm in hell
	with fire
me:	awesome!

	say hi to hitler
	and my fourth grade teacher
Grace:	already did
me:	nice. thanks.

2:04 PM

me:	why hell?
Grace:	not really
	just really busy
me:	i mean, i'm sitting down trying to make a syllabus.
Grace:	when are you back
me:	ahem
	27th
Grace:	oh soon
	Great!
me:	and i teach on the

2:05 PM

me:	get this
	28th
	soonish
Grace:	what are you teaching
me:	did you have an ok bday?
Grace:	yeah
me:	"speech and communications"
Grace:	what's that?
me:	"the art of public speaking"
Grace:	oh
	hilarious

2:06 PM

me:	right
	are you teaching this year?

Grace: well it should be fun

            no

            i'm assistant director

            right now i'm writing the handbook and annual report for the
            writing center

2:07 PM

Grace: it's actually a shitload of work

            more than teaching

            i totally got conned

me: ha

            cant talk further now

Grace: me neither

            lateer

            i love you

me: will talk soon.

Grace: can't wait to see you

me: love to you too.

September 8, 2007, 9:40 am

From: GG
To: LM
Date: Sat, Sep 8, 2007 at 9:40 AM
Subject: Chat with Grace G
mailed-by: gmail.com

9:31 AM

me: me

Grace: yay!

            did you get the pictures i sent you?

9:32 AM

me: dad

Grace: you did?

9:33 AM

me: yes

            did was get

            very

Grace: good

            i'm so glad

9:34 AM

me: it is right

9:35 AM

me: ugh

Grace: i know it's ok

9:36 AM

me: cant i can dont yet

Grace: i know

            but that's ok

            i'm patient

me: i am is good

9:37 AM

me: thing is to much right know

            i love you

Grace: ok

me: lot

Grace: that's ok

9:38 AM

Grace: I love you so much

be patient with yourself

you are doing a great job

it's hard

me: this me right email

Grace: i will write you

me: thank

Grace: Ok

i'll think of a good story

9:39 AM

me: NY

soon

Grace: I KNOW!

are you excited?

— — —

me: lots

Grace: ok love, i'll send you an email

i'm excited too

9:40 AM

Grace: give your parents hugs

and tell them to give you hugs for me

you are my favorite

my favorite in the whole world

Bye!

9:41 AM

me: love

12

In LA I was accustomed to not talking much, and Jonah seemed to be fine maintaining long periods of silence in New York. I appreciated that.

I would write on the bed while he sat at his desk, and for hours we'd keep a comfortable quiet, as if we were each hermetically sealed, even when inches apart. These stretches of communal silence would end with a subtle cue, usually from him. If we looked up at the same time, Jonah would wink or raise an eyebrow, our work would quickly be shuffled away, and the bed would be put to more active use. New York had been demanding for me, and there were many activities that I was incapable of doing. Sex was not one of those things, though. Once it started, the rhythm found itself.

It was an initially awkward conversation to bring up contraception again, since I had been on the pill the entire time I had known Jonah. I was unwilling to take on the increased stroke risk now, but I still wasn't getting my period. My neurologist thought it might be an OB issue, and my OB thought it was a neurological issue. So, we had to be careful in new ways.

Outside the bedroom, Jonah made an effort to initiate social activities we had never done as a couple before. We went on the carousel in Prospect Park, saw a concert in the drained pool on the border of Williamsburg and

Greenpoint, and scored tickets to a game in the Subway Series. Jonah was lighthearted. Sometimes, when he would pass by me in the apartment, he'd take lazy bites at my arms or ears like a grazing ram—*chomp, chomp, chomp.* We were creating a pattern of togetherness, and I was finding a lot of ease in that.

The Girl I Used to Be had complained that Jonah was too contrary and too iconoclastic for his own good. He could never make a simple gesture. Everything had to be categorized, explained—and often diluted—until it fit into his exact dimensions of an appropriate experience. I might have been exactly the same way before the rupture. Regardless, Jonah was becoming more unself-consciously appreciative of me, and more consistent in all of his gestures. I bathed in this devotion.

Of course, Jonah's mood swings were not so easily resolved. They were, after all, part of his psychological makeup. The Girl I Used to Be couldn't help but blame herself when Jonah's disposition would sour, assuming she was somehow the cause. I now saw these shifts completely independent of my own behavior. Though he was being more affectionate with me, he was still unsparing to himself.

One night, he went out drinking with a friend, and when he came home, he started bemoaning the current state of his acting career. He and I had attended a show the night before, from a company he often worked with. A middle-aged reviewer from a downtown paper recognized him in the lobby. She said she hadn't seen him onstage for a while—had he stopped acting? She was provoking him a little, but if I had to hazard a guess, I think she was actually flirting with him in a totally benign way. But this conversation was still gnawing at him.

She asked me if I was just a "flash in the pan," Jonah said to me. And the worst part is: I didn't want to be in that stupid play. If I am being honest, I don't want to be in most plays. Even when work picks up, I probably won't even like the roles I'll be cast in. I'm too smart for this whole acting bullshit.

I hated to see Jonah like this and wished there was something I could do to help. But the more he spoke, the more I heard the eerie echoes of The

Girl I Used to Be. She had been at a similar crossroads, I realized, when she senselessly fretted about why she wasn't cast in more shows in New York, or how her theatrical life might be affected when she applied for grad school, or when she tried to calculate the ramifications of becoming a teacher over a glass of wine with Krass in Paris. Why did she feel she needed to be so definite about everything? Why wasn't she more generous with herself? While she was worrying about her deficits, she seemed to have no awareness of her surplus. This was a woman who could skim a thousand pages a day if she needed to. In addition to being a PhD student, she was also a performer, dramaturg, script reader, theater reviewer, editor, director, and freelancer in the literary departments of Manhattan's most prestigious festivals and companies. She could write dozens of e-mails in an hour. She could memorize a lengthy monologue in less than a day, and when she did, she'd retain it for years. She was the woman often put behind a front desk of a high-powered office, fielding phone calls, welcoming clients, and smiling like the deity of interpersonal communication, able to grow another limb when another duty required it. And she had been just as dismissive of these talents as Jonah was of his. None of this had satisfied her.

I didn't know how to talk to Jonah about this dichotomy, and didn't do much to comfort him, except to offer him my shoulder.

He was still so adaptable. Yes, he hadn't satisfied his ambition, but this wasn't such a dire situation either. Flash in the pan, flash in the pan—it had been such a weird phrase to use because Jonah was only twenty-five years old. This temporary dissatisfaction would probably be the motivating factor in the next steps he would make in his life, and I had every confidence he could undertake those changes.

Jonah dug his head deeply into my collarbone. Maybe this is just a system of failure, he murmured under his breath. Maybe failure is the point.

13

On June 19, I would turn twenty-eight, and my friends insisted on throwing me a dinner party while I was still in New York.

The chef for the night was another former roommate of mine, Stephen, a brilliant theater director. BJ, Laura, and Rachel arrived for dinner at Stephen's house early, with Jonah following soon after. The group was small. Grace had already left for Princeton, and though I had hoped to see Krass in New York, he had already embarked on his yearly return to Paris.

Stephen's directorial career had been incredibly diverse, and he had actually directed everyone in the room, except for his boyfriend. He had directed Rachel and me in *The Bacchae*, so many years ago. But tonight, he was the chef. And he looked like a natural in the kitchen. Long ago, he had lived with BJ, Laura, and me in that dumpy old apartment we shared in Brooklyn, so his current place near the river was a glamorous upgrade. His journalist boyfriend was pouring cocktails, and Stephen was busy putting out some appetizers.

A little *amuse bouche* for everybody, he said.

Can you believe this metamorphosis, Lauren? Rachel asked me. She pointed over to Stephen, who was making leeks and mushrooms in a

Romano sauce to be followed by seared duck in a hazelnut pilaf. This magnificent creation from the guy who used to be obsessed with the crappiest
of all snack foods, she said. Do you remember how he used to hide those
ninety-nine-cent cookies and chips in his sock drawer? And how BJ always
ferreted them out . . .

The memory for this came on cue. But it was a faraway image. In the
foreground, I mainly saw the gourmet cook stuffing endives and truffles
expertly.

Though Rachel had seen me since the second surgery, BJ, Laura, and
Stephen had not, and were eager to find out how it had differed from the
first. Why hadn't I spent more time in the hospital? Had the plates in my
head set off the metal detectors at the airport?

The fact that my aneurysm was being held together with cotton and
superglue was a point of great fascination and discussion between Laura
and BJ. I made a joke about skimping on surgical materials by plundering
the arts and crafts corner of a kindergarten.

Stephen put his knife down in exasperation. I can't believe the way you
guys are talking about this! he said. Especially you, Lauren. This thing that
almost killed you. Could still kill you, God forbid. If this sort of thing happened to me, I promise I wouldn't discuss it. He poured himself a cocktail,
visibly shaken. This conversation topic would be off-limits. Forever, he
concluded.

Oh, come on. You can't really be that surprised that Lauren likes talking about this stuff, Laura said. She was always drawn to the medical and
macabre.

Was I? I asked her.

For sure. Laura laughed. If someone sustained a wound in our old
house, you were the first in line to change their gauze. You'd give me these
unsolicited manicures, and you'd push my cuticles so far down you'd make
my fingers bleed.

So true. Stephen nodded, smiling. When I got back from my trip to
Ibiza with a whole-body sunburn, you picked at it more than I did.

Everyone began to bombard me with details about my past self. Laura reminded me that I left red lipstick traces on every piece of paper in the house, because when it came to blotting my lipstick, I did so regardless of whether it was an important document or not. BJ said that I would sing Ani DiFranco or Italian opera in the shower in the morning while everyone else was trying to sleep. Stephen mentioned the way I would only speak in Spanish when we went to our favorite Mexican restaurant up the road, mainly to impress the waiters. It was agreed that I could be a good time when I was drinking, but occasionally a bad drunk. And much to my discomfort, everyone emphasized that my sexual escapades in that house were never quiet affairs.

My guts twisted in chagrined contrition. I sound like such an asshole, I said.

Hell, no! Laura retorted. You were a weird weirdo, but like all of us. We loved you for it.

And Rachel used this as an opportunity to burst into song, serenading me. *There's no people like show people, like no people I know. . . .*

Dessert was served in a quieter moment. When everyone retreated to the corners of the living room, nursing their coffee or port, BJ snuggled up next to me.

So, he said. What is it like to be back?

It's strange, I admitted.

Mmmhmm. Returning to New York after time away is really challenging because the place never slows down for anyone, he said. When I was in the Peace Corps, I was away for almost two full years, but as soon as I got back everyone acted like I had never left. They waited for me to resume everything as it was before. And they had this image of the kind of person I was, as if they had access to my inner character. People can be so damn sanctimonious. They didn't leave any room for what might have changed in me. I know that I'm not exempt from doing it, but I remember how much it used to upset me.

Exactly, I said.

Yeah, there are pros and cons to having old friends like this. BJ sighed.

It's delightful when they remind you of these amazing things you were part of and managed to forget. But it's hell when they remember things you don't want to be associated with anymore. They can really kill you with embarrassment.

It was an eloquent description of my inner tug-of-war. I thanked BJ by kissing his scruffy cheek.

In this period away from New York, I had found a lot of companionship in books, as I had as a child. But there were limitations to that beyond my language disorder. There were certain things that Laura or BJ or Rachel could provide for me that Helen Keller or Casanova could not—like shared memories, for one. To recall a memory is very often a collaborative event, and you remember different things with different people. My community in New York was playing out a kind of script we had devised together in the years we had known each other. This sort of resurrection had annoyed me when Rachel had tried to engage like this back in LA, but now I was seeing a new value in it. My friends had been maintaining reliquaries of our experiences, and their recollections were actually making some of these traits resurface in me. It wasn't all bad. Maybe my post-stroke changes weren't as dramatic as I had initially imagined, but even if my stroke had reduced me to my basic elements, I was beginning to settle into a form again. And I was surrounded by this incredibly welcoming troupe, who all seemed to be giving me full license to be exactly what I had been and whatever it was that I was becoming now. Nothing could be more generous.

We are conditional beings. No matter how much we want to believe that we are a "certain type of person," we are hugely shaped by our context— what we do and with whom we do it. We are mimics of one another, and we imprint on one another in the deepest of ways. These people at the dinner party had been molding me, as I had been molding them, for years.

If Krass had been in attendance that evening, he would have reminded me that learning was more subtle, more passionate, and more basic than anyone gave it credit for. It was an art. It boiled down to: What do you see? And how does it make you feel?

In Paris, I had been tearing up my heels in this cute pair of white pumps I had bought for the trip. But Krass became squeamish when he saw me pull off some Band-Aids after a day of walking around with him. He admonished me for being so impractical. I fired back quickly, telling him I had seen Parisian women wear the same type of shoe, and there were similar models in shop windows there. He conceded that was true, but these were the type of women who only wore them down the elevator and into the car.

Lauren, you are trying to live two lives inside one pair of shoes, Krass said to me. I respect that. I do. But it is time to come to terms.

Krass wasn't able to be in the room with us, but I felt his spirit then. And although in Paris a year ago he had been talking about an entirely different set of circumstances, his advice had never seemed so relevant. Two lives indeed. It was time to come to terms, whatever that might mean.

14

A few days later, I was getting ready for Jake and Nick's wedding. They were mutual friends of Jonah and mine who had actually gotten married in Canada, but were hosting their reception in a Brooklyn backyard that afternoon. The issue was that I had received an invitation and Jonah had not.

I was applying lipstick in front of Jonah's bathroom mirror, while he sat on the bed, sulking.

I'm sure you can come, I said.

It's not like Jake and Nick don't know how to get ahold of me, he muttered. I'm just surprised. I always thought we got along pretty well.

Just come as my date, then, I said.

I'm not trying to be nitpicky here. I just don't want to be a wedding crasher, either. He paused. There must be a reason they didn't want me there.

Something stopped me. A lurking memory began its synaptic crackling, and though the connection was initially unformed, it started to resurrect when I fused words with those thoughts.

Weren't you involved with a girl from their theater company for a while?

Jonah's eyes widened. That's a really weird thing to bring up right now, he said. That can't possibly be the reason, could it? She and I aren't even in contact anymore.

It had happened in the year before the rupture. During a stretch of time in which I had thought Jonah and I were at our strongest, I would later discover he was not at all monogamous with me. It was BJ who told me first. The girl was in our social circle, and though BJ didn't think relationships had to be exclusive (many of his weren't), he believed in accountability. The fact that Jonah had not openly disclosed the information to me yet was completely unacceptable in his eyes. BJ said, with no small amount of snark, that if Jonah and I were sowing a certain type of garden together, I should also know where he had been planting his parsnip.

After speaking to BJ, I stormed off and immediately confronted Jonah. He didn't deny anything. As always, he was honest to a fault. But this relationship with this woman had become more important than any of his former trysts. He was conflicted.

Is it possible to be in love with two women at the same time? he asked me.

My fury surprised me, and this was one of the few incidents when I raised my voice at him. Had he no sense of tact? Or decency? If he was going to fuck around, I should be the first to know because information like this should never surprise me, and I should never become the recipient of other people's pity. Even though there was an arch sense of sophistication in my verbal attacks on Jonah, it couldn't actually disguise my throbbing sense of betrayal. My mind could allow concepts like confusion or flexibility. But a love shared? That was exactly my limit—something my heart couldn't bear. I broke up with him that afternoon.

But in the course of weeks, or months, this woman somehow disappeared, and I eventually reappeared. My relationship with Jonah did resume. Did he beg my forgiveness and abandon her? Did she leave him and did he return to me after? I still don't remember. It had been one of the darkest periods of our relationship, and it was exactly these moments that Jonah never wanted to revisit with me.

. . .

Still, Jonah didn't see how this old affair should have any bearing on the wedding party that afternoon.

We are all adults, Jonah said. It's all in the past and I don't have any problems with the dynamic among the three of us. He was still fixated on the general principle of his exclusion, and he was complaining that social interactions certainly didn't need to be managed in this way. But Jonah's behavior changed when he shifted his attention to me. When I became his focus, I saw actual concern appearing in his eyes and his voice sanded down all of its rough edges. I guess this whole issue only matters if this matters to you, he said. Does this dynamic bother you?

It was an interesting question. There were certain things about the wedding I felt apprehensive about. Would I be able to keep pace with everyone else in conversation? In what ways would my aneurysm or aphasia come up in interactions? And how long was I expected to socialize? The presence of Jonah's former lover milling through this backyard party had not yet registered on my scale of anxiety at all.

I don't think it bothers me, I told Jonah. Does that change your mind about coming?

You go and have fun, he said. I just think it's best if I stay here.

When I arrived solo at the party, my self-consciousness soon proved unwarranted. BJ, Laura, and Rachel were all at the reception, and being in the company of actors, I hardly had to do anything at all in conversation. I'd forgotten how easy it was for performers to amuse themselves with an inexhaustible talent to self-narrate. When I would ask a simple question at the party, a person would often give a long-winded response, which took the attention off of me entirely. They wanted to talk about their new show at Joe's Pub or their company's touring schedule for the next few months. Some people brought up my medical experiences discreetly, but a few had never even heard about it.

Near the dessert table, I finally glimpsed Jonah's ex-lover, whom the very thought of had once brought so much suffering to The Girl I Used to Be. The other woman was in a yellow dress, drinking rosé in a plastic cup, and tucking a curl of her bob behind her ear. Barefoot in the grass, she looked happy and relaxed. But when she met my gaze, her panicked eyes darted away, her face going through a series of micro-expressions, crunching into dozens of wrinkles and creases, and she was careful to not glance in my direction again.

Surprisingly, seeing her didn't bring up old feelings of jealousy, or flare new ones. If anything, I wished I hadn't brought out that clear discomfort in her. I briefly noted this sighting in my journal, but only mentioned that I got a glass of water after it. Whatever concerns The Girl I Used to Be had about her or this part of my life were no longer my concerns. It was as simple as that.

When I replay this memory to myself now, though, I experience something more fractal, inflected with much more Theory of Mind. It's probably because I'm writing about it. Because now, I am not just thinking about this woman, or even what she might have been thinking about me. I'm doing even more mental division. I am also wondering what was she thinking that I was thinking about her.

What a curious little moment that was. It was left unanalyzed when it happened, but is enriched and changed by examining it now. It is the same anytime we talk or write about a memory—it can launch a thousand ships of thought. It's just a question of whether or not you want to board any of those vessels, and when is it a useful journey. You have to be selective about this sort of thing. I know too well that when a brain doesn't have the right answer, it will fill in a blank anyway; it will simply offer a substitute, and sometimes the possibilities may be fantastic and rich and even insightful, but all too often, it will insert discomfort in places it never needs to be.

15

Jonah's eyes flicked open as I picked up the extra pair of keys on his kitchen table. The midday sun was coming through his curtains, and I had been up for hours.

You headed out? His voice was tender and soft as he rubbed the sleep out of his eyes. I didn't think you'd be going out so often.

Neither did I, I said. But I am finding ways to manage it, and there are still lots of things to deal with here before I return to California.

I'm impressed by the way you've been attempting to do so many things on your own, Jonah said. And you've been succeeding so often, I've been thinking maybe you don't need to go back to LA at all. . . .

Impressed was a wonderfully satisfying word to hear from Jonah, but the second half of his sentiment didn't make any sense.

What do you mean? I asked him. I have to go back—I have my angiogram next month.

Oh yeah, he said. Okay, well, after that, then. You can just come back here. You obviously wouldn't have to pay rent.

It's not just rent. I mean, what am I supposed to do here?

You could do what you do at your parents' house, he said. Keep recovering. Keep writing. You just do it in my house instead.

My affection for Jonah had not waned on this trip; if anything it had increased. But expectations were much more tempered in California. In my parents' home, I helped out with cooking and cleaning and did some assorted errands. Other than that, though, I was able to devote the rest of my time to language. I could read, write, and speak all on my own timetable. There was no urgency for anything because my parents didn't need much from me. But it was clear that Jonah absolutely did.

I should get going, I said.

Then Jonah sat straight up in bed. Why don't you want to stay in New York? he asked. Why won't you let me take care of you?

Oh, Jo. I placed my purse on the floor and sat next to him. I slowly guided his fingers on my uneven scalp, where the screws could still be felt jutting from the skin.

You shouldn't have to take care of me, honey. This is not about another person. Parent. Boyfriend. Whatever. I have got a lot to sort out, and the issue really is time. If I want to keep getting better, I think I need a lot more time.

Jonah let his head prop against mine, and we listened to each other's long inhales and exhales. I looked at the gift Jonah had given me for my birthday on the desk. It was a ridged and ornate conch. He had said he wanted me always to be able to have the ocean at my ears. We both knew there were no ghostly waves inside, and the rushing sound in that "seashell resonance" could be replicated with or without a shell because the echo was produced by the person listening for it. But that didn't make the sound any less beautiful, or the gesture less moving.

When you first arrived, I wanted to convince you how well we could live together, Jonah said. Like a trial run. And didn't we do well?

Better than well, but I still have to go.

I know. Jonah sighed. It doesn't take a genius to realize you're not ready for this yet. And now I'm afraid I'm ruining your final days by talking about you leaving.

You haven't ruined anything, Jo. We're both just trying to figure this out.

Jonah pulled his head away from mine to look at me. Lauren, he said, I just want to let you know that I'm not going anywhere.

This statement confused me at first. *Going anywhere.* Was he traveling soon? Where in the world would Jonah be going? Then, I realized he was speaking figuratively. He wasn't talking about travel, but fidelity. He was saying we could stay together even while we were apart.

Indirectness seemed important to this moment with Jonah, so, although it no longer came naturally to me, I tried to speak to him in this kind of code, too. I said something about not taking "sides" in this game. But I think my message came out garbled even as I was saying it. I wasn't about to pursue another relationship, and I wasn't encouraging him to do so either. However, I didn't know how long we'd be apart. Whatever transpired in our lives away from each other, even if it included other people, I wanted him to know we could still be on the same team.

I wake up in New York, like I do in LA, with soun. But ist is much harder to remember my dreams here. Jonahs body beside me, I wake with a list call citibank. Call landlord.

I am surprised when he brings up the issue of my leaving. I shad thought about it, but didn't want to ruin the last days I'm here—he felt the same. "Before you came, I was ready to have you move in with me but now I think I see now that you need alone. He is disappointed. I didn't expect and prepare much, but instead sure happy finding that we do live somewhat well together.

But what again about leaving. "I'm not going anywhere," he says, endearingly and cryptic. I say "I will not get another side against you," which decoded said "If you find someone or somewhere else, I will not become your enemy. I can't wait for him to wait indefinitely with no known resolutions.

Ever since I was a preteen, New York City was the only place I ever wanted to live. In fact, my mom says this desire began earlier, and she suggests that this interest goes all the way back to my fanatical viewership of *Sesame Street*. But the place required so much focus now, and when my attention drifted (as it often did), crossing a street or in the middle of a conversation, my language would drop out, and I would lose sense of what I was doing and even why I was doing it. The city's pitch and yaw was far too demanding for me. I would have to rehearse conversations before I had them—with the clerk at the bank, the subway attendant, the acquaintance at a party. And though I had planned to return to my grad school to discuss the conditions of my medical leave, I hadn't dared step foot inside. I didn't even call. It would have been impossible to resume the workload of the doctoral program that I was still officially enrolled in. That class I was supposed to be teaching would have to go on without me.

I packed up my stuff in Greenpoint and Jonah helped me sell off all of my furniture on Craigslist. Though I thought about putting the boxes in storage nearby, I didn't know how long I would be keeping them there, so it ended up cheaper to ship them back to California.

My friend Emily offered to help out on the day of the parcel pickup. She had done her level best to look after the apartment when I was away, but it got a lot more challenging when she moved to New Jersey to manage an art gallery. When she met up with me in Greenpoint, it was the hottest day of that summer, made even more stifling since the window air-conditioning units had all been sold. And by the time the UPS guy arrived at my door, he was dripping from his greying buzz cut, sweating through his brown jumpsuit. He started cursing when he saw my tower of packages—16 boxes, weighing 561 pounds. Thirteen of them were filled entirely with books.

The guy started to rail about the "desk jobs" back at the office who hadn't prepared him for this kind of cargo, and, though we had informed him that we would be taking things downstairs as well, he said two little girls in flouncy dresses were going to be as helpful to him as a chainsaw in a prostate exam. Every new parcel he lifted brought a new string of curses that might be mistaken for Tourette's syndrome, if the language wasn't so consciously controlled. And some of the phrases were brand-new ones for me. *Shitdick. Cockjockey. Assbag.* The guy wasn't threatening us. He was exclusively addressing himself to the items he was carrying. Emily and I were bearing this burden too, but for every box we shared, he carried alone. And it was hard not to find his inventive stream of expletives funny.

At the very end of the job, the final box slipped from the man's sweaty hands, falling down half a flight of stairs, and this one he actually kicked the rest of the way to the door. All I could do was laugh. I hadn't noticed the absence of this stuff for most of that year, so why get attached now? Books could take a heavy bruising.

When the man arrived at his van, he hit his absolute limit when he found a parking ticket stuck to his windshield. He began kicking the wheels repeatedly. After all this nut-breaking work? he shouted. You filthy (*kick*) rat-infested (*kick*) cunt-dumpster! (*kick kick kick*)

Although every fragile thing I had placed in those boxes was now broken past repair, I felt a sort of kinship with the UPS man. This city had been an obstacle course for me as well. I approached his open door and asked him if he needed anything. Could I run upstairs and get him an ice-cold bottle of water?

Whatever lady, he said, waving me off and climbing into his bucket seat. You just do me a favor. Next time you lezzies need some help, call FedEx!

As he was pulling away, Emily and I laughed until we wheezed.

Well, that's an elegant New York swan song if I ever heard one, she said. You never know when this city is leaning in for a kiss, or about to give you the finger. Try to tell me you won't miss this.

16

Returning to Los Angeles, I was in a reflective mood. Being around old friends had brought out different parts of my personality, different parts of my language. I could see my thought patterns shift accordingly. I wondered then: If language changes thought, what kind of thoughts are impossible without our full, natural language?

This is the kind of research that Harvard professor Elizabeth Spelke has spent a good portion of her professional life doing. Working in developmental studies, Spelke designed a groundbreaking experiment that dealt with the strengths and weaknesses of language, partially borrowing from a model that began in animal tests, asking how rats behaved in a room in regard to their spatial reasoning and their perception of color.

The rats were deposited in a rectangular room that was all white—white ceiling, white walls, white floor. A bit of food was deposited behind a flap of fabric, and then the rat was turned around and released to find the morsels. The rats weren't searching completely blindly, though. They had a sense of geometric arrangement (they could differentiate between a long wall and a short wall), so they arrived at the target area 50 percent of the time.

Spelke conducted a follow-up experiment, but this time with both human and animal subjects, and added a new element too: a blue wall. Although the rats could perceive direction and color, the blue wall made no difference in their search. The rats and the young children who Spelke included in her study were both largely unaffected by the color change. But, the young participants remained unable to integrate the two separate sets of information (navigation and color) at the same time. They still were finding their target by a large amount of chance.

That is, until the children turned a certain age.

Adults proved to be beyond proficient in the task, and around the age of six, children also become adept at it. They become able to take in the environmental changes and adjust their behavior accordingly. This is when the blue wall starts to matter.

Why could the adults excel, but young children and rats could not?

Spelke and her colleagues (Hermer-Vazquez and Katsnelson) gave a somewhat revolutionary answer. They suggested that language itself might be the missing link. And when I first heard about this study, that suggestion both confused and thrilled me. I had long proposed to Jonah that language was capable of being a unique process of creation, so I needed to know more about their hypothesis.

The team proposed that children were acquiring a certain linguistic aptitude at around age six, in which the concepts of *direction* (left versus right) and *color* (blue versus white) could be analyzed *together*. Spelke suggested that language served as a bridge between these disparate abilities, which were completely self-contained without it, but could suddenly engage with one another when language was inserted into the dynamic. And if that hypothesis was true, language didn't just change the behavior, language itself made those new thoughts possible.

Charles Fernyhough also explores this sort of idea in *A Thousand Days of Wonder*, which chronicles his daughter's first three years of life. When Fernyhough's daughter begins to acquire aspects of language, he seeks to understand what the implications of this new type of communication could be. The question of linguistic relativity comes up a lot. He asks, "Was she finding words for thoughts that had already been there . . . was language translating thought, or creating it?"

This very question lit a fire in me. It is the same one I had asked about myself throughout my language redevelopment. Long after Spelke conducted these experiments and Fernyhough published *A Thousand Days of Wonder*, they were invited to be interviewed together on NPR's *Radiolab*.

The interviewers asked Fernyhough, "What is thought without language?"

"I don't think it's very much at all," responded Fernyhough. He stood by his belief that young children "don't think," at least not in the way he imagines thought. He explained, "If you reflect on your experience, if you think about what is going on in your head as you're just walking to work or sitting on a subway train. Much of what is going on in your head at that point is verbal. I want to suggest that the central thread of all of that is actually language, it's a stream of inner speech. That's what most of us think of as thinking."

Spelke disagreed slightly, saying that Fernyhough might be "exaggerating the role of language here." She called language a "fundamentally . . . combinatorial system." She continued, "Everybody has always talked about how language is this incredible tool for communication that allows us to exchange information with other people," but she added that, "Language also seems to me to serve a mechanism of communication between systems within a single mind."

It's an enthralling proposition and appealed to me on several fronts. In Scotland, when my internal and external language had both become disconnected, my abilities for sophisticated recollection and future planning had suffered, too. And people like Boroditsky, Spelke, and Fernyhough all proposed that language itself could be a source of all kinds of cognitive changes. There is a possibility language may have influenced my Theory of Mind as well. There are many psychologists who insist that it plays a key role in regular childhood development, though there isn't nearly as much research related to language and ToM reasoning after a brain injury. Every time I came across a bit of research like this, I was trying to contextualize myself inside of it. And when it came to Theory of Mind, I had arrived in Scotland a socially adept creature, interpersonally intuitive, but as soon as I acquired a language disorder, I suddenly became unable to understand other people's basic intentions or predict their likely responses. What if language was the common denominator when it came to all of my disorientation?

Most of my skill sets and knowledge base were mainly left intact after the rupture. But these capacities weren't interacting with each other in the easy way they used to, remaining self-contained, isolated. If they were fully formed pearls, they didn't string together to make an entire necklace. And that is why thinking about language in the way Spelke suggests—as a system that facilitates all kinds of other combinations—is so attractive to me. Because if that was true, someone who has lost neurological fluency is bound to feel emotionally disjointed, too.

In my case, I observed that as more vocabulary returned to me, as my grammar and syntax improved, as I became able to use the subjunctive forms in my sentence structures, I was able to navigate through my memories a little more easily. This was also when I started to re-engage in my abilities to understand or anticipate another person's worldview. However, these were just personal impressions, and I am not really in a position to say what is causation or correlation here.

While my language was still very much on the mend, I would seek out any information from people who shared the same condition, even if only on the page. But these accounts were surprisingly difficult to track down. I was never in a language support group, and since the disorder breaks down the basics of linguistic communication, it should go without saying that first-person accounts written by people with aphasia tend to be rare. This was why I paid such close attention to Jacques Lordat.

Lordat had been a well-respected professor of physiology in France in the early 1800s, with a focus on medicine and surgery. Though he experienced his aphasia more than two hundred years ago, his self-reporting is still considered a major touchstone in the literature about the disorder. Oliver Sacks wrote about him, as did Iain McGilchrist. I was thrilled when I first heard about him, and poured over his account, ready to find something in his case that would resemble my own.

But as I delved in further, I was quickly surprised to see that his descriptions of his experience were noticeably different from my own. He writes:

"Within twenty-four hours all but a few words eluded my grasp. Those that did remain proved to be nearly useless for I could no longer recall the way in which they had to be coordinated for the communication of ideas . . . Inwardly, I felt the same as ever. This mental isolation which I mention, my sadness, my impediment and the appearance of stupidity which it gave rise to, led many to believe that my intellectual faculties were weakened . . . My memory for facts, principles, dogmas, abstract ideas, was the same as when I enjoyed good health."

Though Lordat articulates his loss impressively, I found his recollection agitating. I had always sensed that my language, and lack of language, had hugely affected my actual thought patterns. When I saw Lordat write that "inwardly" he felt "the same as ever," I couldn't make sense of that at all. "External" and "internal" speech were inextricably linked for me, and I assumed this was the same with anyone else with aphasia. We all intimately knew the Quiet, didn't we? So I tried to reconcile Lordat's version of this condition with my own, trying to hammer our experiences into the same shape. Was he right, or was I right? Because our positions seemed mutually exclusive.

Later, though, and much more slowly than I would have wished, I realized that things weren't so straightforward. Lordat made it clear that aphasia was not a *thinking problem*, but a *problem transmitting thought*. It was an impressive stance to take at the time, and that viewpoint has left a very positive legacy for those with the disorder.

But I thought, and still think, that aphasia can sometimes be a bit of both those things: a cognitive issue *and* a transmission issue. However, concomitant conditions may strongly come into play here, too. After all, no one can acquire aphasia without a brain injury, and who is to say if another aspect of their injury is producing their symptoms? Also, whether or not people with aphasia have access to their "inner voice" might create a huge variety in the way people experience the condition. It would be a very grave mistake to think that someone who acquired aphasia was no longer knowledgeable or capable. People with aphasia remain chess champions, problem-solvers, financial whizzes, and high-level managers at nonprofit organizations. They can continue to be devoted spouses, parents, and children. They can remain kind or funny. The many manifestations of aphasia can be as unique and various as the people experiencing it.

I mention this because my social group would eventually include many people with aphasia, of all ages and nationalities, including a young woman who had also lost her language at twenty-seven, as a result of an ischemic stroke. Like me, she had gotten most of her language back, which gave me a rare opportunity to have a very fluent dialogue about the issues I had been thinking about for years. And one afternoon, as we sat down over a glass of wine facing the River Thames, I asked about her inner monologue going mute. She had no idea what I was talking about. This had never happened to her. She told me that she had the same knowledge and sense of identity she always had. Like Lordat, she knew what she wanted to say, and the main struggle was that she couldn't express that knowledge.

So what is the most reasonable and fair way to bring up cognitive issues that might come alongside an experience of aphasia? Well, at least in my case, lacking my inner voice for a period of time made a profound impression on me. A word makes an idea concrete, an object that can be grasped and shaped in the hands of the person holding it. A passing perception, or an intuition, can be incredibly complex sensations that don't require any words at all. But these types of mental activities are ephemeral and they don't get so situated in space and time. They tend to be slippery. I often think the strength of language is its exactness, especially when it can communicate ideas that are *not right here* or *not right now*. Language can depict what is no longer visible, or something that has yet to be. And lacking those strong abilities can affect a person's sense of identity. Or mine, at least.

17

As the Fourth of July approached, my family decided to take a trip down to San Diego for the holiday weekend. My aunt and cousins were on a vacation out of state, but they suggested we use their home as a getaway retreat. The brush on the roads nearby remained charred from the fires, but their part of town appeared undisturbed. And to my delight, their infinity pool in the backyard was pristine.

Swimming had been a passion of mine since I was a child. A lifelong asthmatic, it was one of the few sports I could participate in without aggravating that condition. In a recent consult with Dr. Giannotta, I was assured that swimming was safe again and would not affect the incision or intracranial pressure at all. I slipped into the pool immediately after our arrival. I relished the shift of gravity—my head had been a heavy weight for far too long. But there was a new pressure that was building in my mind, unrelated to my brain.

Before I had gone to New York, I had made an appointment with my OB-GYN. I hadn't had my period since the rupture, and I wanted to talk about birth control options, since the physical part of my relationship with Jonah was going to be a part of my time there. The nurse practitioner mentioned something I had never heard of before: an ovulation machine. Most women used the contraption to monitor their periods and maximize their fertility while trying to conceive, but it was a highly sensitive and effective tool. She proposed a somewhat unconventional approach. She said, with some slight reverse engineering, it could also work to prevent conception as well.

Later, as I stood in the family planning aisle at Walgreens, I stared a little uneasily at one of the boxes for these monitors. There was a bald, lily-white baby on the front whose eyes had been visibly enhanced to look highly alert and more attractive to prospective mothers. The box baby's expression was meant to say: I could be your baby! I tried to avoid its Photo-Shopped gaze and ignored the text on the side, which read "not suitable for a birth control method." Sticker shock settled in at the register when the cashier rang me up.

Two hundred and twenty-three dollars?! Aghast, I asked the cashier to double-check. Is this really the price?

The middle-aged Latina behind the counter did her best to sympathize with what she assumed was my situation.

I know it's not cheap, honey, but you are going to love it, she said. I got pregnant the second month I used it!

While I was floating in the pool in San Diego, I started to do some mental calculation. I had taken the device from California, to New York, and back to California again. That meant I'd been using it for forty-five days now. But the icon that indicated peak ovulation had yet to appear once.

Of course, I knew that I was using the machine for a purpose for which it hadn't been intended, and a number of things could be contributing to confusing results and atypical hormone levels. But there was another possibility, too. Maybe the machine was working perfectly, and it wasn't telling me when I was ovulating because there was already an egg very much in use.

Though one of the first things I had asked my neurosurgeons when I woke up from the craniotomy was about possibly conceiving one day, I didn't mean I wanted to have a child any time soon. I wrote extensively about my pregnancy concerns in my journals over the next few days, trying to write myself to any kind of satisfying conclusion.

> *What if I was pregnant? What then? I ~~don't~~ can't imagine raising a baby with Jonah at this juncture—though possible somewhere in the future. So what would I do? An abortion or adoption.*

I had been adamantly pro-choice my entire life, and still felt how important this option needed to be for women. But it was much harder to think of myself making a decision like that at this exact moment. I fretted about what I called *improbabilities.* Improbably, I had survived a ruptured brain aneurysm. Would I be able to force myself to terminate an improbable pregnancy? However, I was also certain that Jonah and I could not embark on parenthood at this point.

So instead, I actually started writing a list, which I entitled:

> *Who could I give it to?*

These were all friends of mine, mainly gay couples, who wouldn't have been able to conceive without dramatic measures. This idea, outlandish though it was, did fall squarely into my category of improbable actions. Would BJ and his new boyfriend ever consider raising a child together? What about Stephen and his longtime partner? Bizarrely, what did not feature on this list was what Jonah's possible reaction might be if I proposed putting a product of our union up for that atypical adoption.

I made it clear to myself that it wasn't out of the question that Jonah and I could actually have a child at some point, but we were currently separated from each other by three thousand miles. Not to mention I was unemployed, and for the time being, unemployable. When I got back to LA, I reluctantly bought a pregnancy test, with no part of me wanting a "plus" sign to appear in the result window.

It was a very long two-minute wait. I placed the test stick on the closed toilet lid and sat on the corner of the cool tub a few steps away. Laura was the only person I mentioned the test to. Jonah could be so opinionated, and I didn't really want his voice to be part of this consideration so early on. He probably would've thought there was absolutely no reason for me to take such a test in the first place. But the doctors I had consulted with told me there was a chance I was still ovulating without menstruating. Now, statistically speaking, getting pregnant before even having my first period post-rupture was highly unlikely. But a healthy girl having two brain surgeries before turning thirty was also pretty unlikely. My entire new life seemed to pulse with unreason; the extraordinary was my ordinary.

One minute passed, but I resisted checking the test window. The strange thing was, in other circumstances, in another life, getting pregnant at twenty-eight would not have been such a source of anxiety. Most of my friends were in their late twenties and wedding invites had been coming in by the handful. I was aware that this was what people did at this age: they got married and they had kids. But I felt I was part of this generation in number alone. My twenty-eight had nothing to do with their twenty-eight. I was close enough to people in these social circles to observe the trappings of their milestones, but far enough away to not even have a whiff of envy. My theater friends tended to delay their childbearing experiences a bit, but twenty-eight was also a big year for a lot of them. And while they were hoping for their banner review from Ben Brantley in the *Times*, I was hoping to master the subjunctive form. I was introducing myself to strangers because they appeared in my dreams, for God's sake! I was not ready to be the mother of anyone's child.

Relief washed over me when the test came up negative.

I called Laura the second I got the results.

Hallelujah, Laura hooted. No babies for you.

That's what everyone says: "Having a baby." But no one is actually having a baby, I said. You are having a human, and they don't stay small for long. Babies turn into tantrumming toddlers, masturbating preteens, self-absorbed college students, and depressive adults.

Preach, Laura said.

The whole idea of making humans is to have your children outlast you, right? I asked Laura. But if your daughter, already living out in the world, has a medical emergency, she'll have to move back in with you for an undisclosed amount of time. You've got to raise her all over again. And this kid will haunt your house and eat up all of your Wheaties. And that's the kind of investment you make when you decide to have "a baby."

Well, that's an effective public service announcement, Laura said. In fact, it's enough to put any sane person off of the idea of breeding for good.

After this conversation with Laura, I cut out the front of the pregnancy test box and stapled it into my journal, with an exclamation point beside it. It was a pleasant reminder of the day's reprieve.

What is past? What is history?
If it is absolutely gone, impossible to access, then it EXISTS ONLY in the minds of the participants.

The strangest part of the documentary is the documents themself.
Recordings. Tapes. Video. Audio.

But even solid, tangible, documents there is only Uncertainty. Each member of the family has a different story, and all of them were involved. All of them were recorded. But they dont ot share a history.

Who do you believe?

I am not a ~~physcist~~ physicist. Or a scientist at all. I cannot understand the terms of an advance or a treat in ~~time tr~~ the science of time travel. But the past, as I know it, is multiple. The past only exists in the individual. Not a point that can be returned to.

Even my story.

The past, as the present, only exists in and by the perceiver.

•   •   •

What is it to love a person with aphasia? Or to be in love with one?

After the rupture, my language rarely matched Jonah's. He exuded what I assumed was the same old fervor and intensity that I had once loved him for, but these days I was always a few steps behind. While we were speaking over the phone, Jonah would arrive at a conclusion in a conversation long before I had even tackled the initial issue, and sometimes he would believe I agreed with him simply because I hadn't been given an opportunity to disagree. In this way, I largely let him dictate the terms of our new relationship, and I doubt that was what he wanted. In fact, he had to do the lion's share of maintaining our dynamic, and I don't think he liked that at all. In his lowest moments, this benign neglect from me would make him feel inessential and unnecessary. Ironically, these were the types of things that he used to complain about in the past phase of our relationship: I had been too sensitive, too easily wounded. Now, I was the one with the "robot voice," though I doubt I noticed this role-reversal in real time. In general, I just found it a little too difficult to confide in Jonah. When we were in the same room together, we could pick up on each other's facial expressions or gentle touch. This intimacy would help us convey or clarify something we felt passionate about. And, in this way, we could rely on the body's grammar. Unfortunately, our bodies were rarely in the same space. The path Jonah and I were on felt uncharted, but we were hardly the first couple to tread it. We didn't seek out examples of other couples who had dealt with these issues of aphasia, but actually there were a number of famous examples. There was actress Patricia Neal and writer Roald Dahl, and journalist Bob Woodruff and his wife, Lee. Later, there would be Congresswoman Gabrielle Giffords and astronaut Mark Kelly. But my favorite aphasic romantic pairing was that of Paul West and Diane Ackerman.

West and Ackerman were both writers, professors, and had published more than twenty books each—fiction, poetry, nonfiction, and literary criticism. This all changed in 2003, when West had a stroke, and subsequently was diagnosed as having aphasia.

West's disorder was more severe than mine had ever been. He had *global* aphasia. Like me, his language was often interrupted, and lacking a fluent flow. Like me, he was bad at producing or repeating words. But, un-like me, he had poor comprehension on top of that. He had difficulty even understanding what people around him were saying. He could only speak a single word for a long while, and it was a nonsense word at that: *Mem.*

Paul West was many years Ackerman's senior. When they first met, he had been her professor. But after the stroke, she became his caregiver. In her book, *One Hundred Names for Love,* Ackerman wonders about a lot of things I imagine Jonah was also thinking about. Ackerman worried that the spontaneity of their love would vanish, eclipsed by the burden of injury. She wrote that she had "never before had to mourn for someone who was still alive," but she did mourn their relationship and "the loss of the word-drenched companionship" that they had lived in.

Though it could have gone another way for Ackerman and West, the story of his stroke became a love story, too. West wanted to write about his aphasia, and Ackerman helped facilitate that for him. And the more he wrote, the more adept he became at writing. And years later, Ackerman was able to write about her side of their aphasic experience. It was a jour-ney of their love, their language, and their love of language. They allowed their shared curiosity to become a propeller taking them into the unknown together.

But in long-term companionship, having a fixed image of the person you fell in love with also makes it a constant struggle to see the person who is in front of you in that minute. Preconceived notions of what *should be* have to be confronted with what *is.* You grow together or you drift apart.

18

Rachel called to check up on me in late July and ended up recounting her recent night out. A self-proclaimed karaoke enthusiast, she was a regular at a few places in the East Village, though she said that she could never exactly think about karaoke the same way after what happened to me in Priscilla's Bar.

Is that rude for me to bring up? she asked.

I told her it was fine, so she continued to talk about the night in Edinburgh, and she did so in such detail it was as if she had been there.

How do you know all of this? I asked her. Laura told you?

Not really, she said. It was all BJ talked about for a while. And there was the video. . . .

The video—I hadn't even thought about the recording since that fateful night. But I knew that BJ had been taping the performance. I had seen him doing it.

Wait, I said to Rachel. You've actually seen the video?

Well, yeah, she said. You haven't?

The very concept made me woozy.

You were doing pretty great onstage, Rachel said. Until your face plant, of course. And if you were going to go out in a blaze of glory, Lauren, you certainly chose a very theatrical way of doing it. Not to mention the song itself. "Total Eclipse of the Heart"?! You couldn't have chosen a better stroke anthem if you tried.

Rachel had watched my collapse, observed the very second the aneurysm had actually ruptured. Somehow I hadn't made the connection that this documentation could still exist somewhere. That it was something I could see myself, if I wanted to.

How did you see this video? I said. And where?

BJ showed it to me, she said. He put it on his blog ages ago.

On his *what*? I couldn't believe what I was hearing.

Don't sound so surprised, honey, Rachel said. We are talking about BJ here. . . .

I wasn't able to take in Rachel's rationale for BJ's behavior, though. My anger was fueled by my embarrassment. It was a highly personal moment and I was horrified BJ had thoughtlessly circulated it in that way. Like my father writing e-mails about me without my knowledge, I felt that posting the video was BJ telling my story without my consent.

But I didn't get as mad at BJ as I had been with my dad. And I didn't stay upset for long, either, probably because I had gotten better at gathering my thoughts and was able to bring up the subject with him right away. When I called BJ, he explained his reasons, and he mainly allayed my concerns.

It's a pretty loose definition of public, he said. No one goes to my blog except me. It's more like a scrapbook than anything else. If you want it offline, I'll take it off. But if you are interested, I can just direct you to the web page yourself. Do you want me to?

Did I?

I wasn't ready to see the video yet, I knew that immediately. But it was an odd proposition. The most seminal event of my life was cued up for whenever I wanted to see it. The next time I reflected on this experience, I wouldn't have to struggle to piece memories together. I could watch it instead of live it. I scrolled down the page, passed the paused video, and read BJ's description, writing some of it down in my journal.

B.j. sent a link he posted on his blog lon ago. October 11, 2007.

The video of the aneursym rupturin—the karooke with Laura.

It is se 15 seconds long thou the player shows me. I will watch it later, but not yet.

B.j.'S below it says "When she fell over, I thought it was funny. When I found out the truth, I subsecquently felt bad."

Posted by Billy J ay 8:44 pm.

0 comments

Labels: Brain, video

19

Through the phone receiver, Jonah was using the singsong lilt in his voice that I enjoyed. He was flirting, but in a relaxed, calming way.

You were so beautiful after the rupture, he said.

But one word struck me, and it broke the spell a bit.

After? I asked him. Why after?

Oh I don't know, he said. You were just so . . . fresh to the world. So open to learn and change.

To learn and change . . .

The phrase disturbed me. Jonah's nudging, which usually felt so playful, could also feel a little predatory. If he liked that I was open to learn and change, would that make him the teacher? Because while I had struggled for words, he had been granted more voice than ever. It was a sensation I couldn't shake recently. And from this statement, I was finding it impossible to determine if this meant that I was actually "the woman who Jonah loved," or someone he would mold into "the woman he could love." Finally, I was finding language for this vague sense of dissatisfaction.

Jonah's stubbornness probably complemented my own in our old relationship, and the ways we were slightly combative with each other—how we could both dig in our heels during one of our debates—must have even been part of the allure. But I didn't operate that way anymore, I simply couldn't. As a result, Jonah had become much more the mouthpiece of the relationship, and my concern now was that he might have come to enjoy that position of power. Maybe he preferred me a little broken?

I didn't express most of this to Jonah, but my inner voice was percolating with these ideas. Jonah intuited that my silence was somewhat fraught.

Lauren, Jonah said gently. This isn't easy for me, either. I'm trying to support you, and trying to make this work. But you effectively live in LA now. I understand why, of course. I'm just . . . I mean . . . How long do you want me to wait for you?

It was a legitimate question, and I tried to answer it honestly.

Six months, I said. A year? I didn't have a good answer for him.

But to be fair, Jonah, I never actually asked you to wait, I said. And there's no way for me to know whether you've been waiting for me or not. . . .

Jonah was startled by my comment. I hadn't meant to question his fidelity, but that was exactly how he received it. His intake of breath sounded like he was on the verge of tears.

What a thing to say. Jonah's voice started to tremble. Of course, of course, of course, I have been waiting. I assumed you knew that, Lauren. And I would continue to wait if you would let me. Jesus, he said. You are not the only person who has changed in the last year.

It was true—I was certain of that. But I am not sure how much that mattered anymore.

I wonder what would have happened if Jonah had offered to come to California then, to start over near me, instead of asking me to return to him. Would that have changed the direction in which our relationship was heading? What if he had asked more questions about my rehabilitation and was less assertive with his opinions of it? What if his senses of integrity and inflexibility weren't so closely aligned? What if he liked my family a bit more? Even a small change on any front could have made a big difference.

I suppose that the extremity of Jonah's moods was a factor as well, but

I am hesitant to say that it was the main one. His unease about where his life was heading was a strong undercurrent in many of his preoccupations, but I had heard similar concerns in our social group in New York, too. The years after college were just an uncertain time for ambitious people.

What was so different in me was that I was protective of, and maybe even a little selfish with, my newfound joy. I would not let my curiosity be eclipsed by anyone else's concerns. And though I had plenty of my own uncertainties in my life, it hardly resembled Jonah's anymore. It wasn't neurotic, it wasn't self-punishing, and it was certainly not defeatist. I appreciated how sincere he always was, but couldn't plunge into cynicism the way he could or the way I used to. Since the rupture, I had been exposed to so many positive and mystifying and terrifying experiences, and death was a lot more present and possible to me. It was a constant reminder not to stray far from things that I valued. If I could die any day, at any time, in any room I was in, I had to make the best of where I was. I didn't need to have a partner who felt exactly the same way, but if I was really going to pair up with someone again, it couldn't be someone who hindered my ways of approaching the world. I preferred comfort to conflict. There were probably a variety of ways in which I could have tried to let Jonah in more. It wasn't very fair of me to exclude him in the way I did, but I really wasn't thinking about how to make any partnership work at that time.

When it comes down to it, I also think Jonah wanted an impossible mix from me. He hoped I would be involved with him and our relationship at the exact level I had been before the rupture. But at the same time, he wanted me to remain wiped of memory regarding our somewhat problematic history. However, memory is what gives us the depth to our experience; it is the way we prioritize the things we hold dear.

A woman without access to her memories, the good and the bad? She would have no reason to invest in anything, or anyone, at all.

20

As the first anniversary of the rupture approached, I opened an e-mail from Krass, who was back in Paris, and I noticed that he had forwarded me a document as well. Above the main text, Krass had written a preface: "Came across this tonight. Perhaps of interest. It is (and was) to me."

As I continued to read, I realized that he had attached a letter *I* had sent *him* a year earlier. It was soon after I had left him in Paris. I had written to him during a low point of the Edinburgh tour, when it had become clear that neither audiences nor critics would be turning out for our production. BJ was irritable, Laura depressed, and my confidence was shot. In addition to feeling like my lack of preparation and experience had let my friends down, I had also recently come across a Fringe publication highlighting the previous year's best shows. The feature article profiled a group of former classmates of ours from NYU, and it was hard not to make quick comparisons. Why had their show been such a success and ours such a failure? What had we been doing wrong? And smack dab in the middle of the page was a large picture of the girl Jonah had had an affair with, the one he thought he might have loved. Her face was shining up at me in smug triumph.

The Girl I Used to Be let her mind reel then, telling herself a story of victimhood.

My self-loathing quotient was pretty high, though I had tried to tone it down a little when I dashed that e-mail off to Krass. The letter was dated two days before the aneurysm's rupture. And it was clear that Krass himself had noticed this dividing line because he had remarked, "From 21 August, 2007, aka another life." And this is what I had written to him:

"sometimes i wonder how it is i got this deep into theater in the first place. an undergraduate degree, dozens (hundreds?) of shows, theater actor, director, reviewer, script editor, dramaturg, and now i'm getting a phd in it? do i really like it that much? i think i am using this degree in many ways simply to sharpen my critical thinking and hone my writing style, that was simply the most complete vocabulary i had to work in/with when applying to graduate schools. wouldn't i rather be writing in poetry in near holyrood or a novel on the rue d st. louis? the answer is an unequivocal yes, but how one makes a career of something like that (without a large parental endowment) is a little more obscure. i certainly enjoy grad school more than being a secretary or a waitress, but the fact that those options are the only ones that seem readily popping to mind is really fairly disgraceful.

this is what is on my mind, between the minutes of 9.09 and 9.36, and may be some of what has been fueling the anxious nightmares from paris to edinburgh."

There was so much about this note that amazed me a year later. The uncertain girl. The girl at the brink of change. Mentioning her writing and her parents, without knowing that her relationships with both were about to alter dramatically. The things that moved this girl, scared her, set her mind on edge would seismically shift in an instant, and would be rendered almost unrecognizable. How could she know what her nightmares were actually portending?

I realized I was so much more satisfied with my life than this girl had been and that much of her dissatisfaction was self-imposed. Now I was working against much more powerful forces, was threatened at much higher stakes, and yet my appreciation and gratitude were abundant. I was much happier now with so much less.

Linguistically, too, there were fascinating aspects in this letter for me to fixate on. The Girl I Used to Be couldn't have been more fluent. In this letter she'd adopted a tone of utter informality, shrugging most aspects of grammar, but even her carelessness showed her mastery. I had to be so much more attentive these days. Carelessness and ease were not something I experienced in my language anymore. But revisiting this piece of writing produced right before the rupture made it easier to review the way I was writing right now:

AUGUST

> *As I continue to work on the book and the journals, I see the fissures of damages. When I write quickly, words change.*
>
> *"A" and "I" become interchangeable. The past ȿtense and the present can switch in the same sentence. Words that sounds like each other "reel" to "deal," "knack" to "knock," materialize without my knowing*
>
> *And strangely, in dialogue, he/she can quickly become me (and I become them) in or around the quotation marks."*
>
> *If I take time to write or review I see them ~~the they~~ "there" ~~the~~ "their" "they're." A pothole on the street. Will it be repaired? Or does the driver need to drive around it always?*

Almost exactly a year after my onset of aphasia, I was still demonstrating aphasic symptoms. In this journal entry, I was detailing them explicitly and describing how they still surfaced every day. But there was also a clarifying self-consciousness in this entry. It was true. I couldn't keep myself from making mistakes, but I also had come a long way from the woman in the Edinburgh hospital who couldn't even know that mistakes were being made. And in confronting my deficits so directly, I was taking charge of my own care, slowly assuming the role I had needed speech therapists, friends, and family members to fill previously. I might never have the linguistic effortlessness of the girl who had jotted that e-mail to Krass, but I was not totally hapless in language either. Not anymore.

I doubt that Krass would have known that sending me that old e-mail was going to spark so much self-reflection. His aim was more direct, practical even. Krass was in Europe again this summer, and this time he had decided to pop over to Edinburgh, to see the Fringe Festival himself. He just wanted to let me know.

Not only was he going to Edinburgh, he would be there a year to the day from the aneurysm's rupture, my near-death anniversary. So I asked him for a favor: to visit Priscilla's Bar. When I called him to make this request, though, he thought it was a little odd.

That's a bit morbid, he said, slightly reluctant to take on the task. Why would you want me to return to the scene of the crime?

Well . . . I struggled to think of a good excuse. I did lose a shoe there. . . .

Uh-huh, Krass said. So this is about replacing a piece of inventory in your closet? Krass was clearly not going to let me get off that easily. You know, Lauren, last I checked there were plenty of shoe stores in Los Angeles. Are you going to tell me what is actually going on here? Or does someone just have a serious Cinderella complex?

I admitted to him then that my motivations were based almost purely on emotion. And actually, that was something he valued and would not dismiss so easily.

What had happened in Priscilla's Bar was not something I wanted to ignore or neglect. I desperately needed a way to mark the occasion of this event, and he might be the only one who would be willing to do it. BJ and Laura probably wouldn't want to relive their traumatic experiences of that day, and I knew my parents would rather forget about it too. Jonah had long ago expressed that I could only celebrate a single birthday. But Krass had already made overtures indicating he was able to appreciate the event more like I did. He had even adopted the language I used about "another life."

So, with no more explanations required, Krass agreed to visit the bar on my behalf. Because he understood what this day meant for me: a rebirth.

21

After living on opposite coasts for almost a year, my relationship with Jonah began its gradual but inevitable dissolution. Every time we'd see each other, we would resume some amount of our intimacy, but it happened less and less and then it stopped entirely. We remained friendly for a long while, though, and he continued every now and then to indulge my desire to hear him read to me.

One particular night in August 2008, he selected *Pieces for the Left Hand*—an excerpt called "Underline Passages."

In the short story, a husband encounters a book of philosophy that profoundly moves him, and afterward feels its pervasive and positive effects everywhere. But at some point, he discovers the book already exists in his house. Not only did he own this book, he had read it already—there were many underlined sections to prove it. How could he have forgotten something so important? Was his sense of the world so faulty? The man starts to doubt everything around him, including his relationship. He and his wife eventually divorce. And while divvying up their possessions, the book appears again. This time, under closer inspection, he sees his ex-wife's name scribbled inside the front cover. It was her book all the time. They were her notes, which he had mistaken for his own.

When Jonah finished reading the story, he whispered, You still awake, Lo?

I am, Jo. It was a good story.

Really? He laughed but sounded like he didn't exactly believe me. You sounded pretty drowsy before I even started. You are telling me you heard the whole thing?

It was a very short story, I said. So, yes, Nosey-pants. I was awake for the whole thing.

Okay, pop quiz. What happened to the couple in the end? Was the conclusion uplifting or depressing for those two?

Hmm, I said. We don't exactly know for sure. It's kind of open-ended. But they have more information about the source of their conflict at least.

You were paying attention after all. I could hear Jonah's smile stretching in his voice. You're learning, Grasshopper.

I gave Jonah an eye roll he couldn't see. I am always paying attention, I told him. But I think both of us might be slow learners.

When does anyone START a true story and when do they teLL it? Like Elizabeth Bennet and Darcy. We hear the story as the villanous Darcy. More history fills in the discrepant knowledge of the <u>story</u>. Time tells him the villains the hero.

A novel begins and ends. The non-fiction story continues with gaps and the fissures.

(For me, there will be details mistakes that Iwwill miss in this book. ~~Prob~~ medical problems, and problems of scientific thinking. But more than that the collating, the rememberig, the <u>re-collecting</u> of this new-time and future time. What what appens after this book is done. The future always the past)

22

August 23. As promised, Krass visited Priscilla's Bar for me ("a dump," he called it; the tone was loving but I knew he meant it, too. He said it was a poor setting to play out the "primary event of your life," adding he believed my mother "chose the FIRST birth with a little more . . . discernment"). It made me chuckle.

Back at home in LA, I was planning my own visit to Priscilla's. I got up, showered, dressed, and sat down on the piano bench at my desk. Pulling my laptop closer to me, I opened the e-mail from BJ and clicked on the link to his blog he had sent months ago.

I read the video's time signature: sixteen seconds. I knew this wasn't the full recording. BJ had warned me that he couldn't find the full-length video anymore, so this would have to do.

The screen had a small, frozen version of Laura and me, arm in arm. The image was grainy, but I could clearly see what I was wearing: my grey-and-white dress with the pockets. There was no reason to be surprised—it had been one of my favorite outfits and was still in rotation. But while getting ready for today's viewing, I had unwittingly put on the same exact dress. Costumed for the performance.

My feelings about what I was doing were still a little uncertain. Few people had documentation of the very second their lives changed forever. Did anyone want to revisit the moment their lives veered onto a different course? But I stopped asking questions and just pressed play.

It all happened too fast. I was up, I was down, and then it was over. I had to watch the video several more times for it to even make an impression. I watched second by second, pause by pause. There was the smile. I am smiling for one and a half seconds. Then the collapse. Laura and I are linked until the moment I slip off her shoulders like a scarf. I disappear from the frame on the word *forever*. And, after that, I can't be seen at all. BJ laughs his unmistakable laugh, his camera shaking quite a bit. The light reflected from the disco ball makes the room look like a purple snowstorm. I am on the floor, but BJ isn't recording the floor. BJ keeps on laughing and Laura keeps on singing and smiling too, looking down at me, waiting for me to return to the song, bruises and all. But things change around second ten. BJ stops laughing. Second eleven, the audio track is going on without Laura's voice accompanying it. Twelve seconds in, the camera shakes, the angle turns, and the recording stops.

Of the sixteen seconds of the video, I could only see myself for fewer than two of them.

I had expected a lot from this recording—a eureka moment. But I didn't see the transition from one person to another. I only saw a fall, and even though I was seeing it from the audience now, I was the only person who knew how important this fall was.

It's every actor's nightmare that something truly dangerous will happen while they are onstage. And the fear is somewhat justified. Fight scenes, duels, and murders are written into a lot of scripts. Performers are taught to disguise the aches and pains they acquire and learn to keep going because the show must go on. But the nightmare scenario is that they might get seriously wounded, too, and amid all of that pretending no one will actually recognize their genuine distress.

What did people think when I fell from the stage? It was a bar after all, it probably happened all the time. They thought that it was just another clumsy girl who hadn't seen the step at the edge of the platform. They thought of the silly American and how foreigners couldn't hold their drink. But they would not have imagined that a dam of blood had broken inside this girl's skull and she was drowning in her own head. A life was seeping out before the audience's eyes, and not one person—not even her friends— realized it right away. The first few times I saw the video, I saw the actor's nightmare come to gruesome fruition.

But as I kept watching, different things came into focus, especially in the final moments. A man off-screen shouts *Oi! Oi!* That's when the hands appear. Laura's hands, the bartender's hands, the strangers' hands—all of them are reaching down for an out-of-frame me.

If I could have chosen the details of my closest brush with death, they wouldn't have included a seedy stage, a gay bar in Edinburgh, or a karaoke night. And I would have selected something a little more dignified than a nose-dive in the middle of a cheesy 1980s power ballad. But it was the role that picked me. Now, I realize that I could have blacked out anywhere. On one of my solo ventures into the streets of Paris without Krass. Or in my New York apartment, when my roommate was out and Jonah and I were taking a night off. Considering all the possibilities available, Priscilla's Bar was not at all the worst place to have an aneurysm rupture. Because if I had been somewhere alone, I almost certainly would have died alone.

There is at least one virtue in falling from a stage—one I never would have thought of before. If you are in front of an audience, there will be someone there to see it. There might even be someone to help you up.

It's difficult to pinpoint the role language plays in our memories—I certainly can't. Ongoing studies of the brain will probably yield fascinating insights into these dynamics at some point. Until that time, I live inside this curious little paradox: my pre-rupture memories are much clearer to me now than they were soon after the aneurysm's rupture, but more time has passed from actually experiencing these events. This means that even though the memories may feel sharper and better defined to me now, other aspects of them are going through the natural process of deterioration.

Writing things down makes this only more complex. Am I remembering an event, or am I actually remembering something I wrote about that
event? There is a strange boundary between recollection and creation, too.

And these days, I find ideas of "the right place" at "the right time"
deeply uncomfortable. To feel faithful, or to sense the working of a kind
of fate in your life, comes with a significant ethical catch, because it is not
accounting for the people in the same situation who didn't have such good
fortune. Why did I live through a ruptured aneurysm when so many in the
same situation don't? Why did I recover so much language when so many
cannot? I know people personally who have worked harder and longer at
this than I have, people who are more intelligent, and probably more de-
serving, who haven't been able to achieve the kind of fluency I have.

All survivors ask questions like these, though it is a peculiar thing to
investigate too much, since it is a temporary situation. I still have two aneurysms in my brain and always will. They will be the cause of my demise
or they won't be, but regardless, I won't remain a "survivor" forever. No one
gets a pass on death.

Still, there is a great indignity borne by some, which is entirely escaped
by others, and this justice is not evenly divided. Money, resources, and priv-
ilege all factor into this inequity. Unfortunately, when well-meaning people
insert a spiritual dimension into conversations about things like this, they
often only complicate the matter. When people say things like "all is as it
should be," or "everything happens for a reason," they tend to unwittingly
highlight the cruelty of these imbalances. And the person administering
these platitudes is all too often the one who has been entirely spared from
this suffering.

With all of that in mind, how do I address a thought pattern that has
played out in my own life, one that I cannot so easily dismiss? Because
when I believe in order, order appears. When I believe fate exists, I see
its workings everywhere. I can't always muster these senses of the world,
sometimes lasting, sometimes fleeting. But I find both of these states of
being equally fascinating. And the fact that my sentiments shift back and
forth, unable to fix themselves on a single judgment, is comforting in its

own way—this is a mirror to the brain itself. It's not that I don't have fear or anxiety or frustration these days. I certainly do. But experiencing how flexible my sense of self can be, and the variety of thought patterns that can play out inside my skull, emphasizes the relativity of it all. That makes it a little easier to shepherd my own thoughts. I try to nourish the ones that are productive and helpful, and starve out the ones that aren't. The Quiet is no longer my baseline, but it is something I try to nurture, and the moments when I connect with it feel sacred, if not sublime.

The human trait of leaning toward faith may simply be a delusion, or a bug in the machine, or an evolutionary adaption for the preservation of our species. After all, it is much easier to live in a world when you can see certainty amid chaos. But if this is only a slight of mind, I'm still grateful for the neural mechanisms that produce it. Human beings meta-cognate—we can think about our thinking. We concoct stories. And when we do that, we get a chance to cast ourselves in leading roles. That is just what our brains do. There are so many systems around us that don't easily follow our personal laws of narrative, or obey our senses of fairness. Yet the brain compulsively searches for meaning, regardless. The fact that a mind, any mind, could produce a sense of faith, or that a person can feel fateful in spite of the churning turmoil that surrounds them, is a miracle in and of itself. What could be more divine than that?

23

I sat down in Dr. Catherine Jackson's lecture hall on the campus of California State University, Northridge, my first classroom experience since I had left my PhD program. Even then the prospect of keeping up with the workload was daunting, and I was right in anticipating that difficulty.

I'd met Dr. Jackson through my friend Betsy's father while I was on a visit to the department of communication disorders. He informed me that Dr. Jackson was writing a book about young stroke survivors. We met at a restaurant soon after, and it was instantly clear that we had many overlapping interests. She wanted to understand more about communication disorders from the patient's perspective, and I craved more clinical information about aphasia, which I had felt disconnected from because of my own linguistic weakness. Dr. Jackson laughed easily and without abandon, and I liked being in her company. It didn't take long before I confided in her about a conundrum with which I was struggling. I felt that though I had rebuilt my vocabulary and skills, I wasn't even close to the level of language recovery I wanted. If a full recovery was never possible with aphasia, when should I consider myself recovered *enough*?

It's a good question, she said. Recovery looks different for different people. For someone who wasn't interested in language in the first place, they sometimes feel like their language is as good as it will ever be in the first months after their stroke. But someone who made their career in words? Who is to say when they are recovered enough?

This statement surprised me, and actually, it completely reframed my own sense of trajectory. This was an internal problem, so I wouldn't find an external solution. I would just have to keep doing what I was doing as long as progress was being made.

During the course of the discussion, Dr. Jackson looked through my journals a bit, and we asked each other questions. The lunch hour came and went, but we were still talking, and we had not at all exhausted our interest in each other. She mentioned that she taught a graduate course in aphasia. She asked me if I might be interested in auditing it.

I accepted her invitation without hesitation, but was nervous, too. How could I possibly keep up?

She promised to make all of the reading materials accessible to me, and attending classes and listening to lectures could supplement the readings if they became too difficult. And I could ask all the questions I wanted, just like any other student. She had only a single condition: I didn't tell anyone that I wasn't a student enrolled in the school.

It's a quirky request, she admitted. But I think these grad students need to see that someone with aphasia can look just like them. You can sit among the class as a student, and then you can later address the students as a guest lecturer.

The idea couldn't have pleased me more.

When it came to schoolwork, the smallest parts of sentences often escaped my first read. Words like *of* and *for* disappeared from the page, which was hugely problematic in scientific texts, because missing them could mean the difference between understanding a cause or an effect. Whenever possible, I bought digital textbooks and enabled their "text-to-speech" functions. I had the books and articles read aloud to me, so I could listen and listen again. I read and re-read. I made prolific notes in the margins. Though it was a lot to take on, it was revelatory as well. I was seeing a personal experience through the lens of academic study, and realizing that issues I'd assumed were unique to my case were not so strange after all. It was like finding some old family album and seeing a portrait of a relative you have never heard of, but who shares a noticeable resemblance to you. I suddenly recognized myself in a much broader context. Dr. Catherine Jackson couldn't possibly have known, but she was igniting a fire inside me, a desire to explore all of the medical, therapeutic, and academic implications of this perplexing condition. It was in her classroom that I started to acquire the skills I needed to engage with this sort of material in the future.

On the final day of the course, I took my place at the podium. I began to read a journal entry from September, approximately one month after the rupture.

First novel. I was 27. Cloud oc
Sparrows
- The ~~right~~ first I do read
a novel, Agagtha Christie.
M, I think. Tried to ~~x~~ try
it 3 pages over and over.

- Words - 3 weeks no
problem. To sleep. The cloud.
After ~~th~~ in

(Seem for ever) When words
back is fever,

I could almost remember writing this, and what I was thinking as I did so. I was recognizing the strides I had made since waking up in the Scottish hospital—from not being able to identify if a book was written by Agatha Christie to being able to actually read the title of a book I had no exposure to previously. Little did I know how much work I had yet to do. Still, I had already experienced a substantial return of my former abilities, and here, even at this very early stage, I was explaining that language wasn't an issue for me anymore. *3 Weeks, no problem,* I had written. Remarkably, and mistakenly, I assumed my recovery was already over.

It was a splintering experience. It begged the question: If I was like that *then*, what must I be like *now*, and what would I be in the *future*?

At Cal State, Northridge, it was my first time speaking in front of an audience like this, but the students looked rapt. And the Q&A went better than I could ever have hoped. I was grateful to discover that other people found these linguistic issues intriguing, too, and I no longer felt I had been wasting my time wondering about them. It gave my confidence a needed push, the confirmation that it might be worth it to keep pursuing my interests in this way.

Afterward, a girl with a shiny mane of hair came up to me. She didn't expect me to remember her, but she explained that we had been at NYU together, in the same small sub-division of Experimental Theater. We worked on a production of *Orpheus Descending*, she reminded me.

It was a Tennessee Williams play, not the Greek myth. But it struck me that the ancient Orpheus was a fitting enough analogy for my post-rupture life.

How utterly bizarre, she said. We met in theater school in New York, almost a decade ago, and then our next encounter is in an aphasia graduate class in Southern California. Only after I've changed careers. Only after you acquired the kind of brain injury that I happen to study now. It's kind of crazy.

I agreed; meeting this way, after all this time, did feel a little uncanny. There might not be such a thing as a "path," but it was in moments like these I felt I was on it. I had been plumbing the depths, trying to resurrect something dear, and in the end, there would be a lot that I would have to leave behind. And like Orpheus, I was bathed in sunlight again, with no going back to where I had come from. But I was a little more sure about what direction I could head toward.

There might be a hidden sense in what initially appears to be senseless, a brilliant kind of order that is invisible to most of us, most of the time. But ultimately, I know that everything doesn't have to happen for a reason. We are more than capable of creating that reason for ourselves.

RETURN TO EDINBURGH

I didn't go to the moon, I went much further—for time is the longest distance between two places.

TENNESSEE WILLIAMS (Tom, in *The Glass Menagerie*)

NOVEMBER 2012

I had always planned to return to Edinburgh, to visit the hospital that had treated me and spend some time in the town that gave me another life. I just hadn't realized how long it would take to get back there—five years and some change.

When I made arrangements for the trip, I thought of the people who had populated the city for me before. BJ and Laura, on our short-lived tour. Jonah, after the rupture. But now BJ was finishing up his final year of medical school at Yale, Laura was working on a farm in Northern Massachusetts with her partner, and Jonah and I had fallen out of touch. We had tried to stay friends, but when both of us started dating other people, a close dynamic was too tricky to maintain.

Jonah wasn't the first person I had loved, nor would he be the last. There was also the man who would become my husband. Sev and I met in 2011, while I was traveling abroad for a friend's wedding in Beirut. Though he had pursued his PhD in Chicago, he wasn't from the US, and he wasn't living there at the time. There were plenty of logistical challenges in the beginning, but he was soon offered a job in London and we moved in together in the UK. Our courtship had spanned three continents, and eventually our son, Isaac, would be born in a country foreign to both of his parents. Though Sev's English is exceptionally good, Armenian is his first language, so I still joke that no one in our household will ever acquire a mastery of American idioms. And after our move, Sev and I tackled a new linguistic challenge of learning all of the new Britishisms, too. But being located in England made it easy to return to Scotland in 2012.

The architecture of Edinburgh's Waverley Station was all glass and stone, full of wide corridors with large swaths open to the elements. There was a dramatic difference, I realized, between the temperatures in Scotland in November and the temperatures in August. As I stepped off my train, I could see every breath I took.

I had traveled by myself, but Alan Paterson was there to greet me. Our families had grown even closer over the years, and their home was much as I remembered it, although Materson had started and finished university by that point. He now had his own place in London. Alan still had the hectic workload of a professor, and Alison had added on even more responsibilities as a teacher and administrator, so their piles of papers were still in every room. The drawers in the kitchen still stuck. And I noticed that the burn mark made by my mother's dropped iron remained emblazoned on their carpet.

Alone on the streets of Edinburgh the next day, I wandered spectral routes. Edinburgh calls itself "The Festival City," and though the Fringe wasn't going on at that time, there was a lively winter fair set up in the center of town. Past the Scott Monument, I navigated through the stalls filled with knit hats and braided necklaces, the air suffused with the smell of sausages and mulled wine. I found my way to the stone stairway that led up the hill in the direction of the Royal Mile. I did eventually stumble upon the theater we had used during the Fringe, but it had been returned to a simple church basement.

Before making the trip, I had been in contact with Anne, my former speech therapist. She seemed overjoyed to hear from me. Though I had expected to visit her during office hours, she said we could meet at the hospital, but after I had caught up with my former nurses and doctors, I could just come home with her and she would make me dinner. I took her up on her generous offer and went to the hospital the day after my arrival.

It was lovely to have an opportunity to meet Dr. Salman, the consultant neurologist who managed my case. Though I had hardly known him in the hospital, my parents remembered him as being inexhaustibly patient with them, responsive to their questions long after my discharge, and he remained in e-mail contact with them for more than a year. Unlike the neuroexperts I had interacted with in the US, he looked directly in my eyes when we spoke and was engaged and reflective with my questions. He was even kind enough to introduce me to the neuroradiologist who had actually operated on my brain. Afterward, I visited my old room with the bed by the window, and handed out chocolates to my former nurses on the ward. Then I looked around for Anne's office. Soon, we were on a bus together, headed to her home. She told me that she'd been so happy to work on my case all those years ago. Many of her patients in the hospital needed help breathing or swallowing and it was somewhat rare that she was able to even start speech exercises with them.

I am so glad you decided to come back to Scotland, she said. Even after such a distressing experience.

It made sense that Anne thought of my circumstances this way, but I wanted to finally set the record straight, and began by taking issue with the word *distressing* specifically.

Actually, I think that whole period after the aneurysm's rupture was much more upsetting for those around me, I explained to her. In fact, most of my memories of the hospital aren't bad at all.

Oh no? Anne was surprised. But you seemed to get so frustrated sometimes. . . .

That was probably true, but I told Anne that left to my own devices, I was usually pretty content. Blissful even. The things that most disturbed my equanimity were often initiated by other people, who were—ironically—motivated by their concern for me.

Anne seemed to consider my comment seriously, and then explained to me that speech and language therapists are often stuck in a very difficult situation. Just because someone couldn't communicate effectively didn't mean that you should speak to them as children. But when you think of them as adults, as people just like you, your empathy engages. You imagine yourself facing such an appalling situation. Sometimes, this thought experiment accurately corresponds with the patient's experience, but then there is the inverse situation, too.

When we *assume* people will feel uncomfortable, we then start to *see* them as uncomfortable without realizing that *we* might be the *source* of their discomfort, Anne said. Expect the worst, the worst can settle right in.

I nodded my approval.

Over dinner, Anne introduced me to her live-in boyfriend, and we crowded around her kitchen table, talking and laughing over her homemade marinara sauce.

Before I left, Anne handed me a Christmas present she had wrapped for me. Inside was a tartan coin purse. The attached card had a photo of the city under a clear sky.

To remind you, she said. It's not always raining in Edinburgh.

A few days later, I went to Priscilla's Bar, though it was no longer called that. And it wasn't a dark hole in the wall anymore. It had been painted a stark white, inside and out. Gone were the cigarette machine and the man in the wheelchair with his dog. The column near the back remained, minus the pole dancers. But the stage was still there. So was the karaoke machine.

I had imagined I could linger in the shadows for a while at this place while I built up the courage for conversation. But, this bright blank box overemphasized the fact that I was the only customer. A woman with long black hair and thick eyeliner was hanging Christmas decorations when I came in, and she sighed as I sat down at a stool. She had clearly been hoping the place would stay empty for a while.

She placed herself behind the rows of booze and asked me what I wanted. I should have thought about this ahead of time, but since I hadn't really come here to drink, I didn't have a preference.

Umm, er. Well. What about you? I asked. What do you drink here?

I don't drink here, she clipped. It's illegal to drink while you're bartending.

She tapped her pale, spindly fingers on the bar impatiently.

The only thing I didn't want to order was whatever I drank the night of the collapse. But I couldn't remember what that was, so I just ordered something I never asked for: a White Russian. The bartender said she would have to look around to see if she had any lemonade.

The only ingredients I knew in a White Russian were milk, Kahlua, and vodka; at least that was the American version. I didn't want to know where lemonade could feature in this mix, and the very idea of it made me suppress a gag. I canceled the order. If my presence in this bar had initially been registered as an inconvenience, I was being upgraded to a full-blown irritation. I blindly pointed at the first Scotch whisky I saw, hoping to stop offending my host. After a few sips, I was able to form the question I'd been itching to ask.

So, I began. Do you know anything about the bar that used to be here?

The bartender said she had bought the place only recently. She was fixing it up and rebuilding the clientele. Why do you ask? Have you been in Priscilla's before?

Relieved that I didn't have to bring it up unprompted, I told her a dramatically condensed version about what had happened in this bar on that very stage.

When I finished talking, the woman seemed to warm up to me a little, telling me that she had a friend who had an aneurysm rupture years ago. Thank God you're still alive, she said, knocking on the wooden part of the bar. But after that brief burst of warmth, she walked away and went back to hanging garlands.

What did I hope to accomplish here? It wasn't even the same place. The staff had turned over. I couldn't ask anyone if they remembered a girl who collapsed in 2007, let alone if they had put aside her shoe for safekeeping. I drained my whisky and got up.

Can I bother you for one more second? I asked the owner. Could you take a picture of me on that stage?

She begrudgingly got down from her ladder again, and used the camera I handed to her.

After she had taken the photo, I glanced at the digital shot. My body looked seriously stiff, my eyes alarmed. I wanted a redo. So I went back on the stage to take another picture, and this one I took of myself, in which I had a little more composure. And as I was climbing back down, I noticed that the platform was only raised a foot from the bar floor. Not a treacherous distance at all. This compelled me to take a photo of the offending step itself.

The bartender became visibly agitated. What on earth are you doing? she asked. What are you playing at?

Confused by the dramatic shift in her tone, I started to stutter.

I to . . . Uh . . . I to . . . told you. Right? Yeah? Didn't I? A p-p-picture of the stage?

The bartender eyed me with suspicion. She said that my behavior had been far too peculiar for her liking. Was I trying to establish a lawsuit? Because if I wanted to sue somebody, she was not the person to sue.

Stunned, I continued to stumble over my words. Though I had gotten so much language back, it slipped when I got nervous. It was clear I was not going to be able to convey the message I wanted to get out: *I am just here for this stage, lady. Me and this step, we have a history.* Floundering more, I tried to explain to her that I was a writer. I just wanted to return to this place, so I could be able to write about it at some point. But I didn't want this part of the story to end on this miscommunication. Only after I convinced her of my actual intention was the threat between us defused, but it was hours before I returned to the Patersons'.

It was late when I came in, but Alison was still up, hunched over the computer keyboard. Her weary eyes glistened as she asked about my night. We laughed over my well-meaning but poorly executed bar visit, and I was starting to head to the guest bedroom when something between the desk and the bed caught my eye.

Are those your books over there?

She said she wasn't sure. She assumed they were her son's because they'd been there for ages. If you saw something in there you liked, she said, you are welcome to take it home.

I moved closer to the stack, which felt like walking toward a mirage because I had glimpsed something that I never expected to encounter again. Gathering dust, it must have been resting on that bedside table undisturbed for almost six years. I had no idea how it left the hospital. Maybe I took it? Maybe someone picked it up for me?

It was *Cloud of Sparrows*.

My present vision started to align itself with the one from my memory, two images next to each other, attempting to fuse. I looked for the birds and the man with the telescope, gazing at points beyond. The colors were intensely familiar, as was the font on the front, and the birds were still in flight. But it was the man who I had the most trouble recognizing. The figure was in silhouette, as he had always been in my memory. But his stance was much more active than I recalled, his right leg bent in a deep, almost ninety-degree angle. And, most importantly, the figure didn't have a spyglass in front of him. He had a sword behind him. The man was ready to strike.

Of course, I was curious what the book was actually about, and whether I would even like it. However, there was something much more to this than the content between its covers. This was a physical object that, until that point, had only existed in my mind. I had plunged into the fog of memory, foraged through an intangible past, and somehow plucked out this article, this matter, this Thing that I was actually holding in my trembling hands. It was not that surprising that I had gotten some of the details wrong. But I had gotten the name right. I couldn't have been wrong about everything.

Over time, I've stopped making large distinctions between The Girl I Used to Be and The Woman I Have Become. Instead, I acknowledged the multiplicities. The person who drank wine on a rooftop in France was (and was not) the same person who opened her eyes in an Edinburgh hospital, who was (and was not) the same person who was writing about those places on a desktop in Los Angeles. Or Beirut. Or London. It is a continuum of selves.

I cannot promise that I am much like the person I was five years ago, or fifteen years ago, or that I will be the same person fifty seconds from now. But I know experiences like this are not limited to people who have had brain injuries. Anytime we talk about our childhood, or any other distant period of our lives, we have to accommodate multiple versions of ourselves—even though we don't sound, or speak, or even think, like these people anymore. My changes were more swift than many. But we all contain these kinds of multitudes.

We are rarely prepared for the next stages in our lives, and we lurch forward into positions we are not equipped for, without the expertise we might sorely need. With that in mind, perfection can never be the goal. But fluidity might be. And sometimes without exactly realizing it, in the process of doing what we are doing, we become the people who are capable of doing it.

Language was both my injury and the treatment of that injury, and in many ways, I have been writing my way back to fluency. I suspect I will continue to keep reaching out for language, even when it falls short. Speech, overt or covert, can be such a gift, but sometimes it is at its best when it isn't being used at all.

How beautiful a word can be. Almost as beautiful as the silence that precedes it.

AFTERTHOUGHTS AND SUGGESTED READING

We lose ourselves in what we read, only to return to ourselves,
transformed and part of a more expansive world.
JUDITH BUTLER

Though at the time of writing this final section it has been nearly ten years after the rupture, I feel that my interest in the brain is still at the level of a beginner. I am absorbed more with its cognitive aspects than cellular ones, more interested in manifest behaviors than chemical reactions. I have taken a couple of courses over the years, but my understanding of neuroanatomy and neuropsychology is rudimentary at best. I see memory as a profoundly social thing—language, too. Both involve a lot of collaboration. We build on one another's language as we build on one another's recollections, and we remember different things when different language is employed.

For a long time, when my family and friends told me stories of our "good old days" together, I couldn't be an active participant in the communal yarns. But now? I have more points of reference and I can take part. I don't just remember the stories, but also remember the tellings and the retellings. Sometimes, I'm able to initiate these stories myself. Language rehabilitation is not a seamless process, and I didn't get everything back. Evidence suggests I never will. Still, I continue to see linguistic improvements. Every year, my speed and fluency get better. It's become easier to recall lines from movies or plays, or banter with a very opinionated friend.

I've been able to tell a joke that had an actual punch line. Many people who live with aphasia report similar improvements, even decades after their injuries. Unfortunately, there is still a widespread assumption in many sections of care that an individual's ability to progress in their language just *stops* at a given time, and many doctors and insurance providers will say that very little can improve six months after the onset of aphasia. This couldn't be further from the truth. Very slowly, people in the neurological community are reconsidering the time frame of language rehabilitation.

I want to make it very clear that my aphasia has never fully gone away and it never will. I also can't gauge how much of my inner speech came back post-stroke. I don't think it is at the level it used to be—or maybe I just won't let that happen—because I don't welcome its many negative and self-defeating aspects. But, in recent years, another voice has joined my linguistic mediations: I have text-to-speech software installed on my computer, my smart phone, and everywhere it is available. This enables every word on a screen to be read aloud to me. I use this function when I read other people's words, but need it just as much for my own writing. Without this compensatory strategy, words on a page can still disappear or warp, and often, essential information is lost in the process. So I type by hand, and I edit by ear. This software is a game-changer for a lot of people with language disabilities and has enabled me to do what I do, but it should go without saying that listening to every word I read and write dramatically increases the amount of time it takes to finish something. It is possible that I might be able to live without this software, but I am also 100 percent sure that I wouldn't have been able to write a book without it.

I mentioned earlier that there aren't a lot of books written by people with aphasia (with some notable exceptions), and this discrepancy carries over into academia since people with aphasia are rarely included in scholarly papers. Their voices are woefully underrepresented in studies, even those dealing with language.

When I was able to access academic reading materials again, I often found myself aligning with people who put forth cognitive models like *linguistic relativity*, which deals with how language directly affects thought. This view of language's role in the brain started to shift when I met more people with aphasia. Once I joined this wider community, I realized that other people didn't always have the same issues that I had. And the more people I met, the more I saw abundant awareness, strategic thinking, resourcefulness, individuality, humor, compassion, and Theory of Mind reasoning, even with little to no language. I had long suspected that my language disorder permeated almost every part of my mind. Maybe it did play that kind of role, but it's also possible I misunderstood that phenomenon even while experiencing it, and my perception of its role infused the rest of my reality. Regardless, I would never want my opinion on linguistic relativity to be the sole reference point for a discussion on how language works in the brain, mostly because I am compelled to write in defense of my own community and its highly unique members. There are so many people with aphasia, and my experiences with this condition should not be assumed to be anything like theirs.

There were many sources I consulted for the writing of this book that didn't make it into this final text, but were still immensely valuable along the way. I want to direct interested readers to them here.

ON MEMORY

In an early draft of this book, Elizabeth Loftus appeared a lot, and though she is no longer quoted in here, her memory research was incredibly influential for me. She has written several insightful books, but I've found some of her journal articles just as revealing, including:

Loftus, Elizabeth. "Make Believe Memories." *American Psychologist* 58, no. 11 (2003): 872.
———. "Our Changeable Memories, Legal and Practical Implications." Nature Reviews, *Neuroscience* 4, no. 3 (2003): 231–34.
Loftus, Elizabeth and H. G. Hoffman. "Misinformation and Memory: The

Creation of Memory." *Journal of Experimental Psychology: General*, 118, no. 1: 100–104.

Loftus, Elizabeth and J. E. Pickrell. "The Formation of False Memories." *Psychiatric Annals* 25, no. 12 (1995): 720–725.

Two other journal articles, from other authors, deserve special mention too:

Garry, Maryanne and Kimberley Wade. "Actually a Picture Is Worth Less Than 45 Words: Narratives Produce More False Memories Than Photographs Do." *Psychonomic Bulletin and Review* 12, no. 2 (2005): 359–366.

Wade, Kimberly, Maryanne Garry, J. D. Read, and S. Lindsay. "A Picture Is Worth a Thousand Lies: Using False Photographs to Create False Childhood Memories." *Psychonomic Bulletin and Review* 9, no. 3 (2002): 597–603.

And Oliver Sacks has written about the limitations of memory, examined from his own life.

Sacks, Oliver, "Speak, Memory." *The New York Times Review of Books* (February 21, 2013): http://www.nybooks.com/articles/2013/02/21/speak-memory/.

See also this book:

Fernyhough, Charles. *Pieces of Light*. London: Profile Books, 2012.

ON NEUROSCIENCE, NEUROANATOMY, NEUROSURGERY, AND NEUROPHILOSOPHY

Costandi, Moheb. He writes the always-fascinating "Neurophilosophy" column for *The Guardian*, and is also the author of *50 Human Brain Ideas You Really Need to Know*. Quercos, 2013.

Diamond, Marian, Arnold B. Scheibel, and Lawrence M. Elson. *The Human Brain Coloring Book*. New York: Barnes & Noble Books, 1985.

Goldberg, Stephen. *Clinical Neuroanatomy Made Ridiculously Simple*. Miami: Medmaster, Inc., 1979.

Luria, A. R. *The Man with a Shattered World: The History of a Brain Wound*. Cambridge: Harvard University Press, 2002.

Marsh, Henry. *Do No Harm: Stories of Life, Death, and Brain Surgery*. London: Weidenfeld & Nicolson, 2014. An entire chapter devoted to aneurysms.

Ramachandran, V. S. *The Tell-Tale Brain*. New York: W.W. Norton & Company, 2011. He includes some fascinating discussion about "mirror neurons" in the brain and how they contributed to the foundations of language, and civilization itself.

Sacks, Oliver. *The Mind's Eye*. New York: Alfred A. Knopf, 2010. He devotes an entire chapter to aphasia called "Recalled to Life."

ON APHASIA

Parr, Susie. *The Stroke and Aphasia Handbook*. London: Connect Press, 2004. Helpful for people living with aphasia and their caregivers.

Tesak, Juergen and Chris Code. *Milestones in the History of Aphasia: Theories and Protagonists* (New York: Psychology Press, 2008), 109.

And as a final suggestion on the topic of aphasia, I strongly recommend readers seek out the writing of Rosemary Varley, currently at University College London, namely because she is one of the very few researchers in the world who works with profoundly aphasiac patients in her linguistic studies. I didn't find her research until the very late stages of writing this book, and have to admit I found her viewpoint on language and cognition initially frustrating because it flew in the face of many studies I had relied on up to that point. But after reading more of her work, and meeting with her several times, I found her incredibly persuasive. Not only that, but she clearly believed in the intelligence and agency of her subjects with aphasia.

She knew that they could think clearly, even if they couldn't speak clearly, and she designed her work with that in mind.

Varley questions a lot of studies that are taken as canon in the academic world. For instance, the Spelke/Blue Wall experiments that I so admired. Varley takes issue with inducing this "artificial" aphasia in people, and complains there were no longitudinal studies. What if people actually got better at the tasks with more practice, and just as little language? She also mentions it has been difficult to replicate these experiments. Varley also doubts the paramount importance of language in Theory of Mind reasoning. She and her colleagues suspected that the linguistic framing in most ToM tests was why aphasic subjects often failed at them. When they devised new tests, actually designed with people with aphasia in mind, their test groups improved in ToM tasks significantly above chance. Below is a primer of her work, but of course, there is much more where this came from.

Varley, Rosemary. "Substance or Scaffold: The Role of Language in Thought." In *Language Disorders in Children and Adults: New Issues in Research and Practice*, edited by Valerie Joffe, Madeline Cruice, and Shula Chiat, 39–53. Hoboken: Wiley, 2008.

———. "Evidence for Cognition Without Grammar from Casual Reasoning and 'Theory of Mind' in an Agrammatic Aphasic Patient." *Current Biology* 10, no. 12 (2000): 723-726.

———. "Science Without Grammar: Scientific Reasoning in Severe Agrammatic Aphasia." In *Cognitive Basis of Science* edited by Peter Camithos, Stephen Stitch, and Michael Siegal, 99–116. Cambridge University Press, 2002, 103, 114.

———. "Reason Without Much Language," *Language Sciences Journal* 46 (2014): 232–44.

Language is a convenient and essential tool to academics and writers. Its descriptive qualities make it immensely alluring, which may be the main reason why so many people (including me, occasionally) tend to believe that language does the heavy lifting in the thought process. But Varley finds the cognitive model of language lacking. She believes language certainly can play a role in our thinking when we're neurologically healthy, and we use it and rely on it because it is efficient to do so. However, Varley has seen that language is not nearly as involved in reason, learning, and decision-making as many people assume. She's been working with people living with aphasia, and she observes how they rely on other inner resources when their linguistic skills have disappeared. For this reason, she believes that language is more like a scaffold. We can see that kind of structure, and since it is the most visible part of the building, we might mistake it for the building itself. But that doesn't make it so.

As far as the language/mind debate is concerned, I think elements of many theoretical paradigms put forth are all valuable in our attempt to answer ever-elusive questions. I like the communicative approaches (expressed by Steven Pinker and the Universal Grammar camp) and the cognitive approaches (represented by people like Boroditsky, Spelke, Fernyhough, etc.). But I am very glad that I was exposed to the *supra-communicative* model that people like Varley represent, too. When we have language at our disposal, we rely on its support, so much so that it feels as if it holds up our entire balance of thought. But if—or when—our language is removed from the facade? Our structure can still stand.

SELECTED BIBLIOGRAPHY

Including supplemental sources

AUTHOR'S NOTE

Basque Proverb

Schacter, Daniel. *The Seven Sins of Memories.* New York: Houghton Mifflin Company, 2001. 139 (emphasis mine), 141.

PART ONE
Chapter 1

Pinker, Steven. *The Language Instinct.* New York: Harper Perennial, 2007. Mortality and morbidity rates for ruptured aneurysms are not exactly static, and somewhat affected by the time of procedure used during the neuro-intervention. The Brain Aneurysm Foundation (www.bafound .org) will have up-to-date statistics.

Chapter 2

More info on aphasia classification can be found in:

Davis, G. Albyn. *Aphasiology: Disorders and Clinical Practice.* Boston: Pearson Education, Inc., 2007.

Chapter 3

Moss, Scott. *Injured Brains of Medical Minds: Views from Within*, compiled and edited by Narinder Kapur 83–84. (Oxford: Oxford University Press, 1997), 83–84.

Morin, Alain. "Self-awareness Deficits Following Loss of Inner Speech: Dr. Jill Bolte Taylor's Case Study." *Consciousness and Cognition* (2008).

Taylor, Jill Bolte. *My Stroke of Insight: A Brain Scientist's Personal Journey.* New York: Viking, 2006.

For more on inner/private speech, consult this overview from Simon McCarthy-Jones and Charles Fernyhough, "The varieties of inner speech: Links between quality of inner speech and psychopathological variables in a sample of young adults." *Consciousness and Cognition* 20 (2011): 1586–1593

Chapter 5

Matsuoka, Takashi. *Cloud of Sparrows.* London: Hutchinson, 2003.

Chapter 6

Basic overview of Theory of Mind (ToM). The "Sally-Anne test" (also called "False Belief Tests") is a famous example of ToM testing, which was partially pioneered by Simon Baron-Cohen, Alan M. Leslie, and Uta Frith in 1985. The test was to establish a child's ability to attribute false beliefs to others (i.e. beliefs that differ from what the child knows to be true). These tests have been conducted extensively in Developmental Studies.

PART TWO

Chapter 1

Ferlinghetti, Lawrence. "Mock Confessional." *These Are My Rivers*. New York: New Directions, 1973.

Chapter 3

Sleep studies and their relationship to memory consolidation are well reported on. This book provides a useful overview:

Carlson, Neil. *Physiology of Behavior*. Boston: Allyn & Bacon, 2010.

PART THREE

Chapter 1

Ruth Lesser and Lesley Milroy write extensively about aphasia and linguistics in *Linguistics and Aphasia: Psycholinguistic and Pragmatic Aspects of Intervention*. Routledge, 1993.

Schuell, Hildred. "The treatment of aphasia." In *Aphasia theory and therapy: Selected lectures and papers of Hildred Schuell*, edited by L.F. Sies, 137–52. Baltimore: University Park Press, 1974.

Szymborska, Wisława. "The Three Strangest Words." Translated by Joanna Trzeciak. Athens, OH: *New Ohio Review*, 2009.

Chapter 5

Jack, Albert. *Red Herrings and White Elephants: The Origins of the Phrases We Use Everyday*. Kent: John Blake Publishing Ltd, 2007.

Chapter 9

Eugenides, Jeffrey. *Middlesex*. New York: Picador, 2007.

Chapter 11

To find a comprehensive overview about working memory and executive functions see: Gazzamiga, Michael S., Richard Ivry, and George Mangun. *Cognitive Neuroscience: The Biology of Mind.* New York; London: W.W. Norton and Company, 2014.

Chapter 13

Emerson, Ralph Waldo. "Nature." *Nature: Addresses and Lectures.* Archived at Ralph Waldo Emerson texts online, http://www.emersoncentral .com/nature1.htm.

For more information on Emerson's aphasia, see: Shenk, David, *The Forgetting, Alzheimers: Portrait of An Epidemic.* New York: Doubleday, 2001.

Chapter 14

Hemingway, Ernest. "A Soldier's Home." *In Our Time.* New York: Scribner, 1996.

Chapter 15

Casanova; Giacomo Girolamo. *The Memoirs of Jacques Casanova de Seingalt.* Translated by Arthur Machen. CreateSpace Independent Publishing Platform; III edition, 2012.

Chapter 18

Whorf, Benjamin Lee. *Language, Thought, and Reality: Selected Writings of Benjamin Lee Whorf.* Edited by John B. Carroll, Stephen C. Lennsen, and Penny Lee. Cambridge: The M.I.T. Press, 1956.

Levinson, Stephen C. "Foreword." *Language, Thought, and Reality: Selected Writings of Benjamin Lee Whorf.* Cambridge: The M.I.T. Press, 2012.

Pinker, Steven. *The Language Instinct.* New York: William Morrow, 1994.

Schacter, Daniel. *The Seven Sins of Memory.* New York: Houghton Mifflin, 2001.

Chapter 19

Since sign language is spatial in nature (and language reasoning and spatial reasoning often live in totally distinct parts of the brain), it might be assumed that deaf people who experience aphasia would do so in a different way to hearing people. But sign language is much more than simple gestures, it is a proper, grammatical language, with all of the identifying characteristics of one (which is discussed at length in Steven Pinker's *The Language Instinct).* In fact, deaf people with aphasia manifest their language deficits in very similar ways as hearing people. There have been fascinating studies done regarding this point. Neil Carlson writes about this in *Physiology of Behavior* (Boston; London: Allyn & Bacon, an imprint of Pearson, 2010) in a section called "Aphasia in Deaf People," (501–502). Oliver Sacks writes about this in *The Mind's Eye* (New York: Alfred A. Knopf, 2010).

Keller, Helen. *The Story of My Life.* New York: Bantam Classic, 1988.

Chapter 28

"6 steps of a Brain Surgery" partially follows the Mayfield Clinic for Brain & Spine "Craniotomy overview" offered at http://www.mayfieldclinic .com/PE-Craniotomy.html.

For more information about the extremely long history of craniotomies (also called "trepanation), please consult: "Ephraim George Squier's Peruvian Skull." In *Trepanation: History, Discovery, Theory,* edited by Robert Arnott, Stanley Finger, C.U.M. Smith. Swets & Zeitlinger Publishers/CRC Press, Taylor & Francis Group, 2003.

PART FOUR

Chapter 1

Dickinson, Emily. *The Poems of Emily Dickinson*, edited by Thomas H. Johnson, Cambridge, Mass.: The Belknap Press of Harvard University Press, Copyright © 1951, 1955, 1979, 1983 by the President and Fellows of Harvard College.

Chapter 3

For more information on phrenology, there was a fascinating article in the Smithsonian Magazine called "Facing a Bumpy History," October 1997, http://www.smithsonianmag.com/history/facing-a-bumpy-history-144497373/

Doidge, Norman. *The Brain That Changes Itself.* New York: Viking Press, 2007.

Freud, Sigmund. *On Aphasia: A Critical Study.* Translated by Erwin Stengel. New York: International Universities Press, 1953, originally published in 1891.

A companion book is Greenberg, Valerie D., *Freud and His Aphasia Book: Language and the Sources of Psychoanalysis*. Ithaca: Cornell University Press, 1997.

Information on localization/neuroplastic can be found in Ramachandran, V. S. *The Tell-Tale Brain.* New York: W. W. Norton & Company, 2011.

Chapter 7

Boroditsky, Lera. "How Language Shapes Thought," *Scientific American* (2011): 63, 65.

Boroditsky, Lera and Jesse Prinz. "What Thoughts Are Made Of." In *Embodied Grounding: Social, Cognitive, Affective, and Neuroscientific Approaches*, edited by Gün R. Semin, Eliot R. Smith, 98–115. Cambridge: Cambridge University Press, 2008.

Pinker, Steven. Quoted in "She explores the world of language and thought" by Barbara Moran. *Boston Globe*: November 18, 2003.

Winawer, Jonathan, Nathan Witthoft, Michael C. Frank, Lisa Wu, Alex R. Wade, and Lera Boroditsky. "Russian Blues Reveal Effects of Language on Color Discrimination." Proceedings of the National Academy of Sciences of the United States of America 104, no. 19 (2007): 7780-785.

Chapter 9

Mee, Charles. *The Bacchae 2.1*, http://www.charlesmee.org/bacchae.shtml: 48.

Shukert, Rachel. *Have You No Shame? And Other Regrettable Stories.* New York: Villard, 2008.

Shukert, Rachel. *Everything is Going to Be Great: An Underfunded and Overexposed European Tour.* New York: Harper Perennial, 2010.

Chapter 10

For a great overview of neurology and the desire to self-narrate, see Gottschall, Jonthan. *The Storytelling Animal.* New York: Mariner Books, 2013.

McGilchrist, Iain. *The Master and His Emissary: The Divided Brain and the Making of the Western World.* New Haven: Yale University Press, 2009.

A lot of what is known about procedural memory owes a great debt to the study of brain patient Henry Molaison, known as HM for many years. A brief overview of his case can be found in: Squire, Larry R. "The Legacy of Patient H.M. for Neuroscience." *Neuron* 61, no. 1 (2009): 6-9.

Chapter 16

Fernyhough, Charles. *A Thousand Days of Wonder: A Scientist's Chronicle of His Daughter's Developing Mind.* New York: Penguin Group, 2008.

Krulwich, Robert and Jad Abumrad. "Words That Change the World." *Radiolab.* NPR (2010). http://www.radiolab.org/story/91728-words-that-change-the-world/.

Lordat, Jacques. In *Injured Brain of Medical Minds: Views from Within*, compiled and edited by Narinder Kapur. Oxford: Oxford University Press, 1997: 71.

McGilchrist, Iain. *The Master and His Emissary: The Divided Brain and the Making of the Western World.* New Haven: Yale University Press, 2009.

Hermer-Vazquez, Linda, Elizabeth Spelke, and Alla Katsnelson. "Sources of Flexibility in Human Cognition: Dual Task Studies of Space and Language." *Cognitive Psychology* 39 (1999): 3–36.

Chapter 17

Ackerman, Diane. *One Hundred Names for Love: A Stroke, A Marriage, and the Language of Healing.* New York: W. W. Norton & Company, 2011.

West, Paul. *The Shadow Factory.* Lumen Books, 2008.

Chapter 21

Lennon, Robert J. *Pieces for the Left Hand.* Minneapolis: Graywolf Press, 2009.

Chapter 23

Williams, Tennesse. *Orpheus Descending.* Dramatists Play Service, Inc., 1998.

Epilogue

Matsuoka, Takashi. *Cloud of Sparrows.* London: Hutchinson, 2003.

AFTERTHOUGHTS / SUGGESTED READING

This quote from Judith Butler was taken from the day she was receiving her honorary doctorate from McGill University, Commencement Speech, May 30, 2013.

ACKNOWLEDGMENTS

There are many challenges in putting together a memoir, and not the least of them is writing about people you personally know, and who were unaware that their words or actions would later be put into a permanent record. For that reason, among others, I want to thank everyone in my life who appears in this book, sometimes under their name, sometimes under pseudonyms. It should go without saying, but I still feel compelled to mention that the remarkable people represented in this story are only fractions of who they actually are outside of these pages.

Especially after my brain aneurysm's rupture, I have been a difficult machine to maintain, and the number of people I really should thank here far exceeds the space provided, so consider this a highly abbreviated list. Thanks to my mother and father for their ingenuity and patience, their creativity and hope, and their massive amounts of love. To my brother, who is one of my favorite people on the planet, who encouraged me to keep writing this book even though it focused on some of the crappiest parts of perhaps the crappiest year in his life. And to Helen Tihista Marks, my beloved grandmother, who passed away soon after my thirtieth birthday.

With her passion for reading, it would have been great to have handed her my own book and hear everything she had to say about it.

With great admiration, I want to thank all my doctors, surgeons, and therapists, because I simply would not be alive without them. I also want to commend the skill and expertise of the team at The Keck School of Medicine, including Dr. Giannotta, Dr. Teitelbaum, Dr. Amar, and Dr. McCleary, and also the team at Western General Hospital in Edinburgh, especially Dr. Al-Shahi Salman, Anne Rowe, my neuroradiologist, and all of the nurses. This huge appreciation equally extends to Dr. Russin and the staff at Justine Sherman and Associates, especially Justine and Alicia.

I do not think there is any way that I can give too much praise to BJ Lockhart, Laura Stinger, Rachel Shukert, and Stephen Brackett—my absolute favorite rapscallions and lifelong friends. Thanks also to Emily Abramson, Betsy Sinclair, Tara Gellene, Kaya Chwals, Shafer Hall, Jason Lew, James West, Albert Lee, Natascha Bussinger, Leslye Headland, Jody Lew, Karen Azarnia, Heather Christian, Catherine Anyango, Alan Chan, Michael Silverstone, Gloria and Russ Kinsler, Darrel Meyers, and everyone from the oatmeal group, my extended family members who appear in this book and those who don't, and to all the individuals mentioned in these pages who I believe would like to remain fully anonymous. Special thanks to the whole Paterson family (and to Abigail Browde for introducing me to them in the first place)—my parents still call them "the angels of Edinburgh." To Virlyn Grant, my grandmother's best friend, the only person who ever rivaled my grandmother's fanatical devotion to libraries, and who has helped keep my grandma alive for me. And to Khanisha Foster, a steadfast friend through it all.

Thank you to all of my teachers and/or readers (too numerous to list!) who have been invaluable to me, but especially: Michael Krass, Sylvia Sukop, Dane Charbeneau, Christine Hauser, Ellen Slezak, Tina Pohlman, Kirsa Rein, Les Plesko, Branislav Jakovljevic, Steven Drukman, Keith Apfelbaum, Laura Cushing-Harries, Kate Britten, Saskia Vogel, and Zia Haider Rahman. Each one of them gave me clarity and insight at many steps along the way, and in some cases influenced me before this book was even imagined. Many thanks to Bryce Howard and Amy Friedman, because no one would have seen this book if you hadn't seen it first. And to Stephanie Douglass, who read many incarnations of my manuscript but also introduced me to my husband, too. She gets some extra points for that!

My gratitude to Catherine Jackson and Stephen Sinclair at the Department of Communication Disorders and Sciences at Cal State Northridge. Also thanks to Liz Seckel and Vivian Chang at the Brain and Cognition Lab at UC San Diego, and to V.S. Ramanchandran, whose work never ceases to amaze me. To the UCL Communication Clinic, Cathy Sparkes, and to Rosemary Varley specifically—thanks for making this book even more complicated in the best possible ways. In my years in London, I was very lucky to have stumbled into Connect, an organization that deals exclusively with aphasic issues, and exposed me to an ingenious model of self-advocacy at work—thanks to all of the staff, volunteers, and members, but especially Alan Hewitt and Anita Foster.

I am indebted to Bonnie Nadell, my extraordinary agent, who believed in this manuscript's potential and was patient as it/I found its/my voice. Also thanks to Millicent Bennett, the brave editor who brought my work in progress to Free Press/Simon & Schuster initially, and to the incomparable Julianna Haubner, who took over this book and always found a few extra hours in the day for me, and shepherded this manuscript to completion. I couldn't have done this without you.

I have received generous support from some wonderful organizations, grants, and residencies. Huge thanks to the PEN Center USA Emerging Voices Program (especially to Michelle Franke, Libby Flores, Aimee Liu, and all of my fellow EVs from that year); the Virginia Center for the Creative Arts (VCCA); VCCA France (with special gratitude to the Francis Heiner and Carole Weinstein grants); Ragdale; the Atlantic Center for the Arts (especially Richard McCann); the Literary Women of Long Beach; the Corporation of Yaddo; and the entire Bread Loaf Community—especially Michael Collier, Ann Hood, Melissa Febos, Carmiel Banasky, and all my fellow waiters. These unique arenas gave me an opportunity to improve my work, be inspired by the art being generated around me, and make so many friends in the process.

My partner, Sev, is my home in this world, who also makes more of this world my home. And thank God for Isaac, who I could not write about much because he only came on to the scene when this book was in its final stages, but who has quickly become the most important character in my life—and I couldn't be more grateful for that.

And one final note to the people who lived the events of the book right alongside me, but do not quite remember them in the exact way I told them. After all is said and done, who says my version is more right? Keep telling your versions exactly the way you remember them. Because I love your stories. I live for your stories.

ABOUT THE AUTHOR

LAUREN MARKS is a Los Angeles native and a New York University, Tisch School of the Arts graduate. She spent a decade in professional theater and pursued a PhD at the Graduate Center at City University of New York. Lauren was an Emerging Voices Fellow for PEN Center USA. She has been awarded grants from the Bread Loaf Writing Conference, Virginia Center for the Creative Arts (VCCA), VCCA France, Ragdale, Atlantic Center for the Arts, and Yaddo, and is an active advocate for those who live with language disorders like aphasia. *A Stitch of Time* is her first book.